Nutritional Considerations in a Changing World

World Review of Nutrition and Dietetics

Vol. 44

Series Editor
Geoffrey H. Bourne, Grenada, West Indies

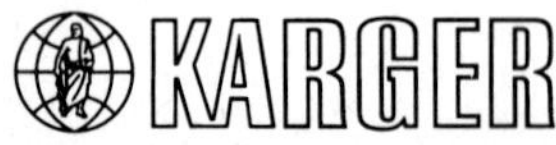

S. Karger · Basel · München · Paris · London · New York · Tokyo · Sydney

Nutritional Considerations in a Changing World

Volume Editor
Geoffrey H. Bourne, St. Georges University School of Medicine,
Grenada, West Indies

18 figures and 41 tables, 1984

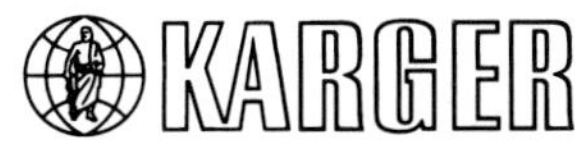

S. Karger · Basel · München · Paris · London · New York · Tokyo · Sydney

World Review of Nutrition and Dietetics

Vol. 41: Aspects of Human and National Nutrition
G.H. Bourne, Grenada, West Indies (ed.)
XII + 260 p., 35 fig., 61 tab., hard cover, 1983. ISBN 3–8055–3591–0
Vol. 42: Nutrients and Energy
G.H. Bourne, Grenada, West Indies (ed.)
XII + 228 p., 27 fig., 44 tab., hard cover, 1983. ISBN 3–8055–3710–7
Vol. 43: Nutrition, Food and Drug Interactions in Man
G. Debry, Nancy (ed.)
X + 202 p., 33 fig., 46 tab., hard cover, 1984. ISBN 3–8055–3800–6

National Library of Medicine, Cataloging in Publication
Nutritional considerations in a changing world/
volume editor, Geoffrey H. Bourne. – – Basel; New York: Karger, 1984.
(World review of nutrition and dietetics; v. 44)
Includes index.
1. Nutrition 2. Food Contamination I. Bourne, Geoffrey H. (Geoffrey Howard), 1909–
II. Series
W1 WO898 v. 44 [QU 145 N9765]
ISBN 3–8055–3837–5

Drug Dosage

The authors and the publisher have exerted every effort to ensure that drug selection and dosage set forth in this text are in accord with current recommendations and practice at the time of publication. However, in view of ongoing research, changes in government regulations, and the constant flow of information relating to drug therapy and drug reactions, the reader is urged to check the package insert for each drug for any change in indications and dosage and for added warnings and precautions. This is particularly important when the recommended agent is a new and/or infrequently employed drug.

Printed in Switzerland by Thür AG Offsetdruck, Pratteln
ISBN 3–8055–3837–5

Advisory Board

Contents

Wld Rev. Nutr. Diet., vol. 44, pp. 1–56 (Karger, Basel 1984)

Nutrition Education in a Changing World

A Conceptualization and Selective Review

Joan Dye Gussow, Isobel Contento

Department of Nutrition Education, Teachers College, Columbia University, New York, N.Y., USA

Contents

I. Introduction

A review of food and nutrition education around the world demands a very different approach than does a review focused on a topic such as vitamin A toxicity. What is needed in the latter is a thorough retrieval and analysis of the published scientific literature; but where nutrition education is concerned there are two major problems in approaching a review in that manner. The first is that the professional literature reports only a fraction of the activity in the field, and even that – as was noted in a recent review of one relatively well-documented sector of the field – is difficult to interpret [*Nestor and Glotzer,* 1981]. Other publications that carry news of food and nutrition education activities, popular magazines, newsletters from various aid groups around the world, reports from clearinghouses or advocacy organizations, provide other – largely anecdotal – information. The sum of all these parts inevitably seems somewhat less than a whole.

This fact stems partly from the other difficulty in the way of doing an academic review of food and nutrition education – i.e. that there is an unclear and even disputed definition of who and what constitutes the field. Does nutrition education include vegetable gardening? Does it include pricing policies designed to influence consumers' food choices or is it properly concerned only with teaching about food as the consumer encounters it at mealtime? Defining the appropriate boundaries of a subject for review always presents problems; these problems are understandably more acute, however, when the topic is as potentially broad as 'food and nutrition education' than when it is – to continue with the original example – as specific as vitamin A toxicity.

Thus the authors have had to acknowledge from the start that it would be impossible (and inevitably misleading) to claim to be doing a 'review' of the field of nutrition education around the world. Certain topics were eliminated from the outset. We will not be discussing the training of professionals whether these be dietitians and nutritionists, physicians or other health professionals, since all these topics have been covered in earlier reviews in this series [*Bosley,* 1975; *Dutra de Oliveira,* 1976; *Fidanza* et al., 1981]. And we have chosen not simply to review the remaining topics that might turn up if one searched the literature (as we have) under 'nutrition education'. Rather, we have chosen to do an *analysis* of the field – looking first at what nutrition education is – i.e. what needs it purports to serve and how those needs have changed over time thereby changing the direction of the field. The major portion of our paper reflects a major change in the field in the last decade, the discipline's growing self-awareness reflected in its practitioners' increased analytical and methodological sophistication.

We will begin the task by looking at the sources of curriculum content, using as a framework *Tyler's* [1950] dictum that the content of any field derives from the needs of the profession, the needs of the learner and the needs of society. We consider the character of programs and practices relevant to each of these, giving special emphasis to the second, since the needs and characteristics of learners, and the nature of the learning process as it relates to eating, have been the source of much program variety and the subject of much recent research and debate. Finally, considering the needs of society, we speculate on how concern about the future affects practitioners' views on the appropriate content of nutrition education today.

II. Defining Nutrition Education

What is nutrition education and how do its practitioners define themselves? The only large organization of nutrition educators, the 15-year-old Society for Nutrition Education based in Oakland, Calif., USA, states that its overall goal is 'to promote nutritional well-being for all people through education, communication and education-related research' [Society for Nutrition Education, 1982]. The Journal of the Society *(Journal of Nutrition Education)* describes itself as 'designed to stimulate interest and research in applied nutritional sciences'. Application would appear to be the relevant word; nutrition educators are interested in applying, for the benefit of people generally, the findings of nutrition science.

What exactly does this mean? In order to get a firm conceptual grasp of what the field is organized to do, we can begin by recognizing that the role as defined above involves relating a very new science to a very old human activity – eating. Nutrition science is no older than the century; humans ate and survived for millenia before there was a science of nutrition or anyone to apply it. Thus it is worth asking why there is any *need* for nutrition education at all. How did people used to learn what to eat?

The answer, of course, is that people survived by the cultural transmission of eating patterns that kept them alive. 'Very few societies', anthropologist *Mead* [1949] told the American Dietetic Association more than 30 years ago, 'have trusted any relationship whatsoever between the individual's natural rhythm, the individual's natural desire to eat, and the diet that he was expected to eat ... Traditionally, in all known societies, ... we have eliminated any natural desire to eat, substituted for it cultural patterns, and enforced these cultural patterns with very heavy sanctions ... This dependence in the past on a culturally imposed eating pattern has kept people alive. We must suppose that in any culture which had too bad a pattern, the people perished ... Thus all the people we find today have a nutritionally viable pattern which they somehow bullied, cajoled, threatened, and persuaded their children to eat. But each such pattern has been based on an empirical nutrition science; if it doesn't include at least the absolutely essential nutrients, the people would not have survived. No one knew what they were doing, no one knew why they ate the things they ate, but gradually, over a period of time, viable patterns have been established' [*Mead,* 1949].

It cannot be assumed that traditional food patterns were optimal, merely that they were compatible with survival through the reproductive years – or they could not have become traditional. It has sometimes been suggested – especially in the popular literature – that primitive peoples have a kind of body wisdom that leads them to seek out and consume the foods they require.[1] Our only evidence regarding human capacity to select a nutritious diet without instruction comes from a single longitudinal study conducted more than 50 years ago [*Davis,* 1928, 1934, 1939]. But the newly weaned infants who performed that feat in *Davis'* laboratory did so under very special conditions. There were no poisons; the foods were neither mixed nor partitioned; they were – without exception – nutritious; finally, nothing was allowed to influence the children except their own appetites.

In asking whether *Davis'* observations are relevant today, it must be acknowledged, to begin with, that such freedom from outside influences exists hardly anywhere. Moreover, instinct would not work unless, as *Yudkin* [1981] has suggested, humans confined themselves to foods their neolithic ancestors would have recognized; the food environment in which instinct might function effectively could not contain anything but 'whole' or 'natural' materials since nature could not have equipped us with selection mechanisms useful in discriminating among not-yet-invented chemical mixtures. And even neolithic children would need to be protected from consuming poisons; *Davis'* infants exhibited none of the neophobia that appears to protect other omnivores like rats from consuming lethal quantities of unfamiliar substances [*Davis,* 1939; *Rozin,* 1976]. Thus it is clear that in the environments from which most humans have actually selected their

[1] The suggestion that people 'instinctively' know what to eat was given widespread public visibility in the USA in 1980 when a newly appointed Secretary of Agriculture discounted the need for nutrition education with the observation that hogs could balance what they ate if offered a basic ration with a protein supplement, and that people were surely as smart as hogs.

diets, children and adults survived not on body wisdom but on cultural wisdom. They followed the traditions of their group.

In recent decades, these traditional food patterns have begun to be very rapidly modified not only in developed countries but in every part of the world which is not wholly isolated from technological civilization [see e.g. *Szczygiel,* 1974]. This has seriously complicated the eater's task. Hunters and gatherers knew and ate a surprisingly large number of different living things. Pastoral herders and more sedentary agriculturists probably made choices from a smaller number of foods. Yet contemporary eaters who have considerably less time and mental space to devote to food acquisition and preparation than did their predecessors must attempt to make wise choices from many more items – as many as 12,000 in a large US supermarket [*Molitor,* 1980]. Some of the most attractive of these did not even exist in grandparents' or parents' generations, and many of them bear an obscured, remote and/or tenuous relationship to foods that might have been gathered, hunted, herded, or grown.[2]

Meanwhile, because technology has made it possible to manipulate foods' sensory properties to make them richer or sweeter or saltier or more colorful at will, the tastiness and appearance of foods no longer informs consumers of their respective nutritional worth. We can no longer use what *Leiss* [1976] has called our 'craft skills' to decide what is fit to eat. We have so fully separated palatability from nutrition that unlike other animals we are no longer assured of getting what we need by simply eating what we want [*Yudkin,* 1978]. In short, humans need nutrition education because in most countries of the world, for the first time in human history, large populations of children and adults are being exposed to attractive food products which are neither biologically nor culturally familiar.[3] This set of circumstances has altered our view about the maleability of diets. Food habits may

[2] *Pelto* [1981a] has commented on the recent growing dominance in anthropological thinking of 'behaviorist-materialist' theories of human behavior, which emphasize the impact of the material environment on behavior, over the older 'ideational' theories which emphasize the 'causal primacy' of cultural ideas. It is worth noting that a theory which posits the importance to behavior – including food behavior – of the material forces which surround individuals may seem increasingly 'correct' simply because the cultural ideas whose seeming power underlay the 'ideational' school have been overwhelmed by rapid change.

[3] The Australian aboriginals provide a number of contemporary examples of the negative impact of 'modern' foods and 'civilized' food practices on peoples whose food patterns are well adapted to a harsh environment [*Hamilton,* 1971].

Table I. Profile of nutrition-education activities in 201 nutrition programs in developing countries

Program aspects	Percent using or including
1 Target group	
Mothers	90
Fathers	20
Other relatives	24
Schoolchildren	35
Influentials	15
Entire community	28
2 Medium	
Demonstrations	79
Group classes	75
Individual counseling	62
Radio	23
Television	14
3 Frequency	
Daily	31
Weekly	33
Monthly	33
During health visits	36
4 Site	
Home	43
Village	55
Health center	64
5 Topics covered[1]	
Weaning foods	77
Balanced diet	73
Pregnancy diet	71
Lactation diet	70
Diets during illness	48
Food preparation	67
Food storage	48
Kitchen gardens	54
Hygiene and sanitation	75
Weight-chart interpretation	52

[1] Not all 182 programs providing nutrition education reported topics covered.
Source: *Austin* et al. [1978]

be hard to change in the direction desired by nutrition educators, but they are not, as was previously believed, generically hard to change in the face of environmental discontinuities.

Out of the preceding analysis it is possible to derive a logical answer to the question of what nutrition education is and why we need it. Given that humans no longer know how to choose foods at least partly because traditional food environments and routes for communicating traditional food-related information have been overwhelmed by technologically induced change, then nutrition education is a way of replacing folk wisdom – about how to acquire, prepare and consume foods that are good to eat – with wisdom obtained in some other way about how to acquire, prepare, and consume foods that are good to eat. And since we now have scientific knowledge about relationships between food composition and nutritional health, our teaching about foods can, ideally, be even better than that which would have been transmitted by tradition.

This insight may help explain why the need for nutrition education was evident so early in the USA, a cultural 'melting pot', whereas such education has only begun to seem urgent in developing countries in the last few decades as traditional cultures broke down under the onslaught of modernization. *Zeitlin and Formacion* [1981] note that it was in 1950 that the report of the Joint FAO/WHO Report Committee on Nutrition first emphasized the importance of nutrition education in health programs [FAO, 1950]. By 1958 the same Committee considered education 'a necessary part of practical programs to improve human nutrition' [FAO, 1958]. Increasingly during the 1960s, as *Zeitlin* and her colleagues point out, nutrition education received a level of priority equal to that of other development activities – no longer was it seen simply as an adjunct to curative health programs. Indeed, when the American Public Health Association surveyed 180 low-cost health delivery systems in developing countries, they found that some sort of nutrition education was included in 88% of them [*Karlin,* 1976]. More recently, the Harvard Institute for International Development [*Austin* et al., 1978] found that 91% of 201 developing country nutrition programs included some nutrition education (table I).

We have come now to a very heuristic question, one that leads to an examination of how the task of food and nutrition education can best be carried out. If nutrition education is – in the broadest sense – a way of teaching which foods are good for people to eat, then on *what basis* ought people in various regions of the world make choices about which foods are good to eat?

III. Nutrition Science as the Basis for Food and Nutrition Education

One answer to this question – the one that seems obvious at first – is that when nutritionists speak of foods as *good,* they are referring primarily to their nutritive value and very secondarily to their practicality and attractiveness. A food is good if it provides essential nutrients, is locally available, and can be put into a locally acceptable food pattern. Whether a food is *good* can thus be very largely determined by analyzing the food and by analyzing human nutritional needs.

The field of food and nutrition education, seen from this vantage point, is structured as a kind of pyramid in which the relevant knowledge is produced at the top by the nutrition scientists. They discover the important relationships between bone synthesis and vitamin C; or the factors that affect iron absorption from bread; they learn what is going on in cells and molecules. These biochemical details, these complexities of intermediary metabolism, are communicated through various professional levels toward the broad base of the pyramid which is made up of the general public. As the knowledge works its way down, the content becomes more and more dilute and a good deal more general (citrus fruits contain vitamin C; vitamin C prevents scurvy) *but it does not change in fundamental character.* Underlying everything that is taught is the root knowledge about nutrients, their presence in food and their functioning in the body.

This kind of approach to nutrition education – one that begins with the needs and interests of the discipline of nutrition science – has had widespread support arising from a number of sources. Science is prestigious (as education itself once was) and the closer science gets to the purely quantitative, the more certainty it appears to possess and hence the more authority it is granted. This hierarchy of prestige has had an effect on who is readily accepted as a nutrition educator in the USA. Many food scientists practice nutrition education, although they are not necessarily required to have studied human nutrition or to have had training in educational theory. On the other hand, concern has sometimes been expressed over allowing those formally trained in education but not in nutrition science (that is school teachers) to teach the public how to eat wisely. The scientification of food has also been encouraged by the fact that nutrition educators have traditionally been women who – in male-dominated societies – needed all the prestige they could get. Hence those who wished to use their knowledge of food and people professionally have hesitated to suggest that there were things about food (e.g. who controls its availability; how it can be palatably prepared) that were at least as important for consumers to know as its nutrient content.[4]

Certain sectors of the food industry have also supported the notion that nutrition educators should limit themselves to providing consumers with accurate information about food composition, human nutrient requirements and the relationships between nutrients and health [*Gussow,* 1981b]. A definition of *good* based only on nutrients gives endorsement to a number of highly processed products fortified with the essential nutrients that assure their *good*ness.

Although nutrient-centered assumptions underlie much nutrition education, perhaps the best known example of an entirely nutrient-based approach in public education is the program of nutritional labeling in the USA. The program evolved in the 1970s out of the recognition that the large variety of items in the market and the complexity of their composition made it difficult for consumers any longer to apply a simple food grouping system in meal planning (one well-known nutritionist was fond of asking in which food group a frozen spinach soufflé belonged [*Mayer,* 1971]). Consumer advocates, regulators and some nutritionists pushed for a standardized labeling format showing macronutrient composition of the food and its content of eight micronutrients as a percentage of a federal standard derived from the United States Recommended Dietary Allowances; and shoppers were to be taught by nutrition educators how to get the most nutrients for the dollar while balancing their diets [see e.g. *Ross,* 1974].

[4] The withering away of 'food as sustenance' concerns in the profession is evident in the trend in the USA to eliminate departments of home economics, either by changing their names – e.g. human ecology – or by fragmenting them and allying nutrition with either health sciences or biochemistry. Other evidence of female professionals' fear of being tarred with the 'food' brush can be seen in the defeat of a resolution (in the face of strong support for all other resolutions) offered at the 1982 Annual Meeting of the Society for Nutrition Education. The resolution proposed that the Society change its name to the Society for Food and Nutrition Education. Although it went down to defeat for a number of reasons, one of them certainly was the concern expressed by a speaker at the Resolutions Hearing that we had to lose the 'home ec' image and that nutrition professionals were having enough problems without being associated with food and cooking. *Kolasa* [1981] reminds us, however, that 'in its early days the field of home economics focused on the interdependencies and interrelationships of families and environments' and that the development of nutrition along single discipline lines led nutrition educators to forget 'the ecological perspectives of their field'.

Even before the system was put into effect, some of its supporters worried that nutrient labeling might enhance the apparent value of heavily fortified foods and might mislead consumers by focusing attention on packaged products rather than on fresh unpackaged produce such as vegetables and fruits which were unlabeled [see e.g. *Briggs,* 1973; *LaChance,* 1973]. From the standpoint of nutrition education it was probably even more important that the system was too complex to be useful. Consumers do not appear to have made use of nutrient labeling to significantly alter their food selections [see e.g. *Friedman,* 1972; *Jacoby* et al., 1977; *Tyebjee,* 1979].

None of the above is meant to suggest that the facts derived from nutrition science are an inappropriate basis for nutrition education, merely an insufficient one. The issue is not whether sound nutrition knowledge is important before one undertakes to teach people how to eat. The issue is how much of what part of that knowledge is useful to those doing the eating, and what else is there that consumers need to know in order to eat wisely?

IV. Nutrition Education for the Learner

As we noted earlier the content of any educational enterprise usually derives from one or more of three sources: the needs of the learner, the needs of society, and the needs of the discipline [*Tyler,* 1950]. An educational approach based primarily on nutrients clearly expresses the interests and needs of the discipline. That is, nutrition educators teach nutrients because that is what the discipline of nutrition is about and that is what we have taken the trouble to learn and think others would profit from knowing. But teaching based on nutrients does not necessarily take into account the needs of learners or of society.

How would nutrition education change if we focused on the needs of the learner? Education about foods seems in order, since the learner's contact is not with nutrients but with foods. But if learners need to know which foods to eat, how do we decide what to tell them?

The appropriate answer to that question will depend on the nutritional status of a given audience, the nature of their food supply, and the context in which nutritional health is sought. Since nutrition education has been longest formalized as a discipline in the USA, that country provides an interesting illustration of the close relationship between the message and the changing nutritional environment. In the USA at the turn of the century when poverty and malnutrition were widespread, it was necessary to teach people how to upgrade the quality of their diets by adding more protein and calories so that children could benefit from schooling and adults could be productive workers. Indeed, as early as 1908, a Dr. *Emerson* of Boston developed a 'nutrition class' method where underweight children were encouraged to compete with each other in weight gains [*Whitehead,* 1973]. The results were so spectacular that *Emerson* was invited all over the country to train people in his methods of encouraging weight gain. With the discovery of the importance of vitamins and minerals during the 1930s and 1940s, the task of nutrition education changed – people were taught to add 'protective foods', fruits and vegetables, to their diets, along with the calories and protein.

Today, however, circumstances have changed again; the average resident of the USA currently eats twice the recommended protein allowance, seldom experiences deficiencies of the major vitamins and minerals, and has a 30% probability of being overweight. For the majority, therefore, there is no longer a need to gain weight, but to maintain or lose it; the challenge is not to avoid nutrient deficiencies so much as it is to avoid such apparently nutrition-related degenerative diseases as heart disease, diabetes, cancer and hypertension.

The experience of other developed countries is similar to that of the USA. Figure 1, which shows the intake of various macronutrients in relation to GNP, illustrates the fact that dietary patterns tend to reflect relative wealth. This is an intranational phenomenon too; throughout the world, it has been suggested, people can be divided into three populations – the affluent, the rural poor and the urban poor [*Davidson* et al., 1979; *Den Hartog,* 1981]. In the less developed countries, even as the growing middle and upper classes begin to experience the nutrition-related problems of affluence, other groups – the rural and urban poor majority – suffer from malnutrition due to lack of adequate food. In Tunisia, for example, adults at higher occupational levels suffer from obesity and high cholesterol levels, but the greatest nutritional problem on a numerical basis is malnutrition among preschoolers [*Forbes* et al., 1979]. The nutrition education needs of this malnourished majority will obviously be far different than those of the affluent minority.

Yet simply acknowledging that the messages must be different depending on the income of the population involved does not in itself help a professional decide just what those messages should be. An example may be clarifying. The Australian aboriginals are generally recognized as a group

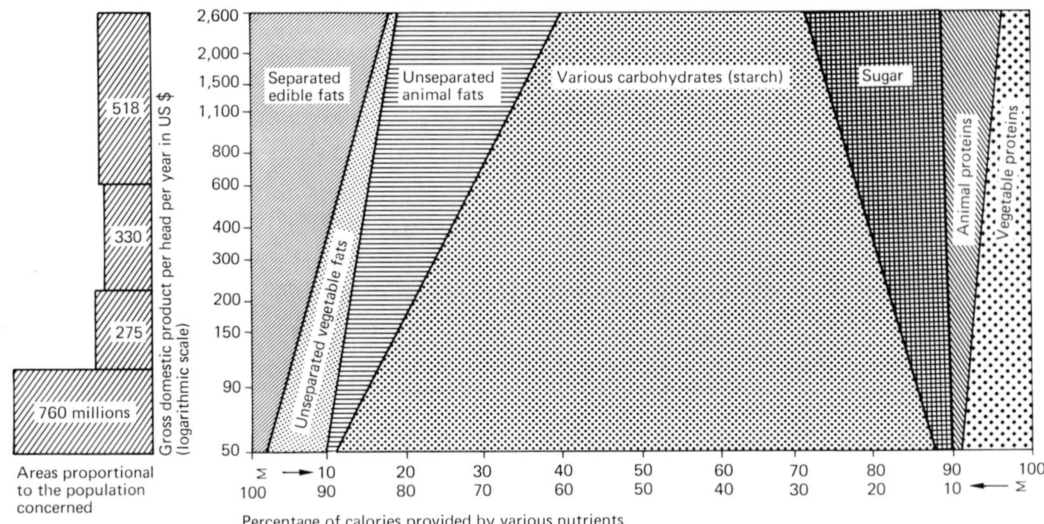

Fig. 1. Calories derived from fats, carbohydrates, proteins as percentage of total calories according to the income of the countries (1962). WHO/FAO energy and protein requirements. WHO technical report series No. 522, 1973.

nutritionally (and culturally) impoverished by their contact with a transplanted European civilization. How should their impoverishment be ameliorated? At the Australian Conference on Nutrition Education [Commonwealth Department of Health, 1981] the nutritionist from New South Wales reported on a series of activities directed to aboriginals in her state. These included encouragement of breast-feeding and use of an electrolyte solution to reduce malnutrition and gastroenteritis among infants and young children, the distribution of food parcels for pregnant and lactating women, and the promotion of fruit and vegetable gardens [*Harding,* 1981]. The nutritionist from the Northern Territory focused on the development of a framework within which problems related to the food chain could be understood from both aboriginal and nutritionist points of view. Foods, whether from the store or from the bush, were classified in patterns meaningful within the aboriginal tradition; food selection was taught on a color basis which made sense in the aboriginal scheme. The 'translation of science to social or cultural terms was based on the existing belief system and not merely simplification' [*Shelley,* 1981].

Faced with essentially similar populations, two nutritionists in different settings chose to focus their attention quite differently in planning nutrition education programs. On what basis are such choices made? That question, which underlies much current analysis and debate in the field of nutrition education, provides a focus for the remainder of this review.

As was earlier suggested, perhaps the most remarkable change in the field of nutrition education in the past decade is the extent to which its practitioners have begun to professionalize the field meeting with each other at conferences and workshops, not merely to report on programs but to raise systematic questions regarding goals, methods, appropriate theory bases and boundaries of content [e.g. *Olson and Gillespie,* 1981; *Sims and Light,* 1980; *Brun,* 1983]. One of the perhaps most fundamental of the questions being raised has to do with appropriate intentions or goals for nutrition education.

V. Choosing Goals for Nutrition Education

When those involved with nutrition education attempt to articulate their goals, they express a variety of stated intentions. At one extreme are those for whom nutrition education means simply providing persons with the knowledge and skills necessary to make their own decisions about nutritional matters. At the other extreme are those who assert that their goal is to change, shape, or maintain desirable eating behaviors [*Contento,* 1983; *Zeitlin and Formacion,* 1981]. These apparently very different goals derive from different notions of human nature and of the process of behavior change.[5]

The former derives from a framework that may be called cognitive-gestaltist. It emphasizes the uniqueness of the individual and the importance of inner cognitive experience such as thinking or insight in learning and behavior. In the USA this framework is represented by the humanistic school of thought, by the work of such psychologists as *Maslow* [1968] and *Rogers* [1969], and by terms such as 'self-actualization' or 'student-centered learning'. Education is seen as being the expansion of self, the release of the inner nature or tendency for good, and the steady increase in a learner's

[5] For a fuller description of the relationship between theories of human development, theories of education derived from them, and the practice of nutrition education, see *Contento* [1983].

self-acceptance, autonomy, and power to shape the environment. In the developing countries this framework is represented by the work of *Friere* [1970]. *Friere* is also interested in humanization, but he emphasizes the overcoming of external oppression through 'conscientization', i.e. the arousing of a person's self-concept through a 'liberating education'. In this sort of educational experience the authority-dependency relationship normally found between teacher and learner is replaced by a situation in which teachers and students become jointly responsible for a process which challenges all the participants to reach a greater capacity for critical reflection and intervention in their world.

When used as a basis for nutrition education, the cognitive-gestaltist framework posits that people are basically good, rational, and able to make free choices, and that if they are given information relevant to their lives in the context of a liberating education, they will adopt those behaviors that are healthy and self-actualizing. Many nutrition education interventions and curricula are based – explicitly or not – on this framework. Thus in one study in the USA, 'discovery learning', designed around games and activities, was used with high school students [*Spitze,* 1976]. A similar strategy was used in the Philippines to facilitate villagers' choice of a development activity involving food raising [*Clark,* 1979]. *Friere's* work also formed the basis for planning nutrition education in a community in northeast Brazil [*Drummond,* 1975].

In contrast, the idea of nutrition education as directed behavior change derives from a behaviorist framework and builds on the writings of psychologists such as *Watson* [1913] and *Skinner* [1953]. This school posits that behavior is not determined by an autonomous inner being but by the environment. More specifically, behavior is provoked by environmental stimuli and maintained by other stimuli, which are (or which appear to the learner to be) consequences of that behavior (called reinforcements, contingencies, or rewards). Thus behavior can be changed or shaped as desired by the application of appropriate stimuli or reinforcements. *Skinner* [1971] rejects autonomy-oriented or self-actualizing practices in education because he sees their claims as an illusion. People are *not* really free anyway, he argues: 'to refuse to control is to leave control not to the person himself but to other parts of the social environment'.

When used as a basis for nutrition education, this school of thought suggests that people are not actually free to adopt healthy eating behaviors when there are so many forces in society – including very sophisticated food advertising – which provoke and reinforce unhealthy behaviors. Healthy behaviors can only be developed, according to this view of human nature, through the use of behaviorist principles, i.e. through setting up appropriate schedules of reinforcement for learners. Behavior modification has been used by nutrition educators (and others) principally in the treatment of obesity [*Coates,* 1981; *Stunkard and Penick,* 1979], but it has also been used in a few situations where tokens and rewards were employed to bring about increased vegetable consumption by children [e.g. *Ireton and Guthrie,* 1972]. The behaviorist framework has been especially valuable in providing a methodology that has been used extensively in research [e.g. *Birch,* 1980; *Galst and White,* 1972; *Schacter,* 1971].

There is an underlying tension between these two contrasting goals of nutrition education; on the one hand, we acknowledge that eating behaviors – healthy or otherwise – are voluntarily chosen by people in light of their own life situations. On the other hand, we are committed as nutrition educators to 'promoting the nutritional well-being of people' – a task that may well include changing behaviors identified by current scientific knowledge as health risks. It has been suggested that this dilemma could be resolved if we sought behavior change as a goal only for those who already have such chronic degenerative diseases as diabetes or hypertension, or who are at clear risk of developing them. For the public at large, so the argument goes, the goal of nutrition education should involve no more than the dissemination of relevant information so that people can decide for themselves which foods to eat.

Zeitlin [1977], in discussing nutrition education around the world, argues that these two goals should be viewed as complementary and that the degree of choice exercised by the community or individual should depend on the type of nutritional decision being made. During a diarrheal epidemic, for example, the reasons for oral rehydration should be explained, but rapid modification of the behavior of withholding liquids is required in order to save children from dying. On the other hand, 'whether to sell eggs for cash or give some of them to the children is a choice only the family can make' [*Zeitlin and Formacion,* 1981]. Yet if the children in a family were suffering from malnutrition we would, as nutrition educators, surely want that family to give some of their eggs to their children rather than sell them all – and we are less than honest if we do not acknowledge that.

This tension – between educating and propagandizing [*Moore,* 1978] – is not unique to nutrition education but underlies all of schooling. We seem to have decided that it is acceptable to propagandize about matters that society as a whole has agreed are important for people to learn – e.g.

the three Rs. That is, it is permissible, indeed desirable, to aim for behavior change if the new behaviors sought are the ability to read, write and do arithmetic. We are less sure just what it is we expect of the high school civics teacher, however. Certainly we want him or her to teach students how a country's government works, and certainly we want students to learn the information on both sides of issues. However, surely we also want students to learn to behave in a socially and politically responsible manner.

Where nutrition education is concerned, the tension between the goals of producing changed behavior or simply providing information for individual decision making is given vivid expression in a recent statement from the US Council for Agricultural Science and Technology (CAST). 'Since *freedom of choice* in the selection of foods is part of our way of life, nutrition education is a high priority issue because the public must be provided with the information that will *encourage good nutritional practices*' [CAST, 1976 – emphasis added]. Assuming that 'freedom of choice' is the underlying goal, the question then becomes: what information is to be provided so as to enable people to select among foods? It is clearly not possible – to take the extreme example of the USA – to inform even a relatively literate population about the amounts of 60 or so nutrients (as well as about the many non-nutritive substances that may affect their health) in each of 12,000 food items, and to provide this information in a form that will enable individuals to make intelligent food choices on their own. If nutrient education involving a dozen or so nutrients on food labels is too complicated to be useful, food labels involving 60 or so nutrients would be even more uselessly complex. However, the decision to leave out some pieces of data and include others inevitably imposes a value on the information retained. Omitting information on the percentage of calories supplied by refined sugar or saturated fat in a product, for example, implies that these facts are less important in making food decisions than are the facts presented on the label. On the other hand, displaying the information that a given product contains 100% of the RDA for several nutrients may imply that the product is highly nutritious.

Selection of content *always* occurs, and always communicates implicit lessons – a fact well illustrated by examining the simplest teaching devices nutrition educators use. These are the various semi-official food grouping systems that classify foods into categories according to the nutrients they contain and recommend specific numbers of servings from each group [see e.g. *Ahlström and Räsänen,* 1973; *Hertzler and Anderson,* 1974]. The food grouping systems used in the developed countries have tended to put heavy emphasis on animal products, reflecting traditional affluent eating patterns. In the USA, for example, the Basic Four Food group system (meat, milk, fruits and vegetables, grains) was long dealt with as if it were merely a convenient teaching tool, and as such was used without objection in government nutrition education activities for 40 years. That it carried an implicit message became evident when questions were raised about the Basic Four's heavy emphasis on animal products in light of the country's major health problems. When an alternative guidance system (The Dietary Goals) that suggested reducing intake of animal foods, sugar, and salt, was proposed [Staff of the Select Committee, 1977], objections began to surface over government 'interference' with consumers' free choice. As *Truswell* [1980] has noted, since these messages 'Have major negative items, anyone embarking on nutrition education is likely to meet lack of interest from politicians, anxiety or delay by civil servants, apathy from the medical profession, a tough counter-attack by the producers and processors of the food(s) you think people should eat less of, and confusion or indifference from the general public'. The Dietary Goals and the more official Dietary Guidelines [Nutrition and Your Health, 1980] which followed them are actually part of a growing body of developed nation dietary advice aimed at preventing disease and promoting health [*Molitor,* 1980]. Instead of focusing on food groups, the recommendations involve reduced consumption of some food categories (fats, sugar and salt) and increased consumption of others (e.g. fiber).

In the developing countries, there has been a move toward greater reliance on local food grouping systems and less on imported systems such as the US Basic Four which was even less appropriate in many of the countries which adopted it than it has begun to be in its country of origin. *Zeitlin* [1977] notes that the most common food grouping system in the developing nations uses three food groups: protective foods, body building foods and energy foods. An alternative four food group system has also been proposed consisting of a staple or starchy food category, and three other categories made up of foods that provide extra energy, protein, and vitamins and minerals [*Abrahamson* et al., 1977]. *Zeitlin and Formacion* [1981] have criticized this system as providing false reassurance about the nutritiousness of the starchy staple, an objection which – whatever its merits – emphasizes once again the observation with which we began: every system, however simple, and however objective it is intended to be, has a series of decisions and assumptions built into it.

Some selection of content must occur in all nutrition education, and in that selection process the curriculum designer or educator inevitably expresses his or her assumptions – implicit or explicit – about which pieces of information will be important and useful to the learner. 'Educating' is thus not possible if what is meant by that word is giving all the facts and nothing but the facts. Such dispassionate and unselective fact giving may appear theoretically desirable from the point of view of the discipline, but it simply does not exist in practice.

Moreover, from the point of view of learners, not only must some selection be made, but the criterion of selection must be to provide learners with 'the understanding, skills and motivation necessary to promote and protect their nutritional well-being through their food choices' [*Ullrich,* 1979]. Once having set out this criterion, we are back to acknowledging that nutrition education inevitably involves information and activities which (so we hope) will affect people's behavior in a way deemed nutritionally desirable.

VI. What Nutrition Education Works?

What kind of education produces and maintains eating behaviors conducive to the long-term health of learners? This, of course, is a question that the profession has grappled with for decades [*Swope,* 1962; *McKenzie and Mumford,* 1965; *Whitehead,* 1973; *Tepley,* 1973]. But in a remarkable and very recent burst of activity – reflected in workshops, conferences and reviews of the literature that express the profession's growing self-awareness and sophistication – nutrition educators have begun to seek ways of learning not just *what* works, but why and how [*Auerswald and Gergely,* 1981; *Brun,* 1980a, b, 1983; Commonwealth Department of Health, 1981; *Enelow and Henderson,* 1974; *Hambraeus,* 1980; *Levy* et al., 1980; *Nestor and Glotzer,* 1981; *Olson and Gillespie,* 1981; Rethinking, 1980; *Santos* et al., 1981; *Sims and Light,* 1980; *Sims and MacNeil,* 1980; *Sinclair and Howat,* 1980; *Zeitlin and Formacion,* 1981].

In 1965, *McKenzie and Mumford* reviewed the published literature about nutrition education around the world and were able to find only 22 research studies in which objective evaluations were included. 17 of these reported a positive change after nutrition education and five reported no change. The reviewers concluded that in the nutrition education studies reported until that time success or failure seemed to depend 'on the methods used, the personalities involved and the circumstances prevailing in the area ...' 'However', they continued, 'we are not, as yet, in a position to isolate these factors more clearly ... partly because so few evaluated studies have been done ... and partly because the purely technical devices for use in evaluation have not been fully developed' [*McKenzie and Mumford,* 1965].

In her more comprehensive review of nutrition education around the world between 1900 and 1970, *Whitehead* [1973] examined in detail several dozen studies (out of more than 100 that she located) that provided evidence as to whether or not the intervention resulted in improved dietary habits. She concluded that nutrition education was a factor in improving dietary habits when learners were involved in active problem-solving with respect to their own nutritional problems, when an integrated community approach was used, and most importantly, *when the methodology employed was designed with changed behavior as a goal.* One of the threads that ran through *Whitehead's* review was the discovery that the most successful approaches to behavior change were those advocated by theorists, such as *Dewey* [1902] and others, who emphasized the importance of the active participation of the learner in the learning process. Thus, for example, the group decision method of *Lewin* [1951], in which participants made a public commitment to behavior change, was more effective than the 'telling' of nutrition. *Whitehead* [1973] also urged that there should be serious research into the methods and techniques of nutrition education. Improving the food choices and nutritional status of those in developing countries was particularly crucial, she felt, since there 'economic productivity is positively correlated with nutrition status and total health of the population' [*Whitehead,* 1973].

In the decade-plus since *Whitehead's* review, there has been an upsurge of activity in the newly emerging field of nutrition education research. Such research is not necessarily intended 'to answer questions about the scientific merit of the message content per se, but to design appropriate messages for target audiences, and to determine the most effective methods for message delivery within given contexts' – i.e. nutrition education research is interested in 'the *process* of nutrition education' [*Sims,* 1980a, b].

A 1981 report of the US Office of Science and Technology Policy (OSTP) viewed the field as concerned with: '(1) Studies of dietary practices, food consumption patterns and their determinants including such areas as: (a) nutrition knowledge, attitudes, beliefs and factors that influence changes in behavior as they affect actual food consumption patterns and practices;

(b) development of theories, models, and methods with which to study these issues, and (c) barriers to dietary adequacy. (2) Studies of methods for informing and educating the public and professionals about nutrition, health, and dietary practices, and research to develop strategies for informing the public about food nutrition, health and dietary practices' [OSTP, 1981].

A review of the proceedings of a number of conferences held to address these issues over the last 5 years [*Brun,* 1983; *Olson and Gillespie,* 1981; *Sims and Light,* 1980], taken together with recent reports and journal articles, indicates that nutrition education research has become increasingly sophisticated as it has begun to make use of relevant theories, concepts, and methodologies from a variety of related fields. In learning how to study the determinants of dietary behavior and to develop techniques that can improve or maintain desirable eating practices, nutrition educators have begun to draw on a number of theories previously utilized in such disciplines as psychology, sociology, communications, education, economics, consumer research, social marketing and community organization.

The theories that have been most used are those from the fields of social psychology and communications that contain elements from both the cognitive/self-actualizing school and from the behavioral school. These theories are especially useful to nutrition educators because they attempt to provide explicit and systematic conceptualizations of how both the perceived social context and internally derived motivations influence behavior. That is, these theories do not simply describe who acts how and where; they attempt to explain *why* people (i.e. learners) act the way they do. Since the theories also suggest strategies for promoting behavior change, they are useful to nutrition educators in both developed and developing countries. The application of these theories in nutrition education has been described in detail elsewhere [*Coates,* 1981; *Contento,* 1983; *Hochbaum,* 1981; *McGuire,* 1980; *Yarbrough,* 1981] but for purposes of subsequent clarity it is worth briefly reviewing some of them – involving attitudes and attitude change, persuasive communication and decision-making, and social learning.

Attitude change theories postulate that people are troubled by inconsistencies – between their attitudes and new knowledge, between their attitudes and those of significant others, and between their attitudes and their actions – and will attempt to restore consistency. In theory, then, behavior change can be brought about by changing people's attitudes. Attitudes may be changed by opinions or beliefs which can, in turn, be changed by persuasive communication. This is the so-called KAB or knowledge-attitudes-behavior model.

Persuasive communication focuses on *senders* who choose *messages* which they communicate through *channels* in order to influence *receivers.* Not all receivers are affected by a message or innovation, however. Trial adoption will precede full-scale adoption and some persons will likely adopt before others so that innovation diffuses slowly through a community.

Decision-making models, in essence, propose that people choose among behaviors on the basis of some kind of cost-benefit analysis of the consequences of each choice. Thus the Health Belief Model [*Becker,* 1974] suggests that whether people choose to adopt a particular preventive health behavior will depend on: (1) their perception of the threat to them represented by some illness or condition; (2) their benefit-minus-barriers analysis of the advantages of taking that particular action to alleviate the condition, and (3) various cues to action coming from internal sources (e.g. a stomach that hurts) or external ones (e.g. nutrition education). The Behavioral Intention Model [*Ajzen and Fishbein,* 1980] suggests that behavior is best predicted by a person's behavioral intention which is in turn dependent on that person's attitude toward a given behavior and what he/she perceives as the behavioral norm of significant others in his/her social environment.

Social learning theory, like the above theories, recognizes the importance of cognitive function in determining behavior, but emphasizes the role of the environment (reinforcements or contingencies) in changing or maintaining behaviors. According to social learning theory [*Bandura,* 1977] behavior change is best brought about by using *all* sources of influence simultaneously: environmental variables (stimuli or reinforcers) can be manipulated to produce and maintain change; cognitive training in problem-solving or self-management skills can be provided; change can be further facilitated by giving the individual opportunities to practice various target behaviors and experience their reinforcing value.

Finally, social marketing theory proposes that the principles and techniques useful in marketing products can be effectively applied to social change programs 'to increase the acceptability of a social idea or practice in a target group' [*Kotler and Zaltman,* 1971]. Understanding the consumer is central to the creation of the right *product* backed by the right *promotion* and put in the right *place* at the right *price.* It must be observed that in practice both research and intervention studies tend to use techniques derived from *various* theories.

While at first glance all these theories may appear unrelated to practice in the real world, especially a real world in which malnutrition dominates, closer inspection reveals that they have great heuristic value both in analyzing the underlying causes of particular nutritional practices and in developing appropriate strategies for changing behavior. If, for example, one's concern is with why a mother does not add fish to her malnourished infant's weaning food, or why an affluent person will not reduce his intake of high fat foods, these theories suggest factors to be investigated – factors such as individuals' attitudes, health beliefs, or benefit-minus-barriers considerations. Or again, if one is designing programs to encourage women to breast-feed or to cut down on salt, these theories suggest alternative strategies that may be useful – persuasive communication aimed at attitude change, or skills development based on the principles of social learning theory.

Investigation into the role of attitudes and beliefs in determining dietary behavior is going on in Australia [*Baghurst* et al., 1980; *Bell* et al., 1981; *Worsley,* 1980], in Canada [*Sullivan and Schwartz,* 1981], in the USA [*Sims,* 1978], and elsewhere. Many of the relevant studies were recently reviewed by *Sims* [1980b]. The research suggests that the relationship between knowledge, attitudes, and behaviors is quite complex. One of the studies, for example, suggested an attitudes-to-knowledge-to-behavior linkage rather than a knowledge-to-attitudes-to-behavior one [*Sims,* 1978]. Others have proposed that attitudes and behaviors continuously interact with each other [*Kelman,* 1974]. *Zeitlin and Formacion* [1981] therefore suggest that nutrition educators should try to influence both simultaneously, and provide many suggestions for how change in attitude and behavior may be brought about, especially in developing countries.

Though little nutrition education research has been based on the Health Belief Model, its usefulness in predicting whether mothers will follow physicians' instructions about breast-feeding has been studied [*Morse* et al., 1979]. Likewise, the Behavioral Intention Model has been studied for its usefulness in the design of a program to increase breast-feeding among low-income women [*Kaplowitz and Olson,* 1983]. The two methods have also been compared for their ability to predict whether people will participate in an immunization campaign [*Oliver and Berger,* 1979]. Social learning and related theories have been primarily used, in research studies, to investigate weight-loss strategies [e.g. *Mahoney and Thoresen,* 1974; *Coates,* 1981], but they have been much less extensively used in research than in the design of interventions.

VII. Non-Formal Nutrition Education

The theories described above have been widely utilized in a variety of non-formal settings where their usefulness in improving our ability to bring about behavior change has been explored. While we can do no more here than cite a few illustrative examples, numerous projects are described in such sources as the guide to nutrition education by *Zeitlin and Formacion* [1981]; *Leslie's* [1977] review of mass media projects, the *Project Profiles* of the Clearinghouse on Development Communication [Clearinghouse, 1982], the report of the Meals for Millions Conference on teaching nutrition in developing countries [*Shack,* 1977], the publications of the International Nutrition Communication Service, the proceedings of the various conferences listed earlier and – as we indicated in our introduction – in newsletters from various aid organizations and other fugitive sources.

A. Mass Media

The relevant concepts and theories from the behavioral sciences have been used in mass media campaigns in developed and developing countries. Examples of the former are the Stanford Three-Community Study and the Food for Thought Project in the USA [*Fortmann* et al., 1981; *Smith* et al., 1981], the North Karelia Project in Finland [*Koskela* et al., 1976] and the 'Life Be In It' campaign in Australia [see *Emery,* 1981]. Examples of the latter are the Mass Media Nutrition Advertising Campaign in the Philippines [*Cook and Romweber,* 1977], the Food in Life Campaign in Tanzania [*Hall and Dodds,* 1977] and the Nutrition Mass Communication Project in India [Clearinghouse, 1982]. Although the theoretical considerations underlying these campaigns are similar in developed and developing countries, the content of such projects and campaigns always reflect the great differences in access to food and in the nature of the nutritional problems being addressed.

For example, the Stanford Three-Community study was designed to reduce cardiovascular risk through modification of dietary, smoking, and exercise behavior. The dietary modification aspect of the campaign was directed at *reducing* intake of saturated fat, cholesterol and total calories to a level that would achieve and/or maintain ideal weight [*Fortmann* et al., 1981]. The campaign was based on persuasive communication concepts and made use of TV, radio, newspapers, billboards, and pamphlets distributed by direct mail. Results reported at the end of 2 and 3 years showed that modest but significant changes in dietary (and smoking) behavior had been brought about by the mass media intervention. One population segment also received face-to-face instruction, using techniques such as self-observation, modeling and token reinforcement derived from social learning and related theories. The results showed larger and more lasting changes in a greater variety of behaviors when both approaches were used [*Meyer* et al., 1980]. A follow-up study involving five cities has been initiated to test further the usefulness of the communication-behavior and social marketing frameworks in health education. This study will emphasize putting greater reliance on local community organizations [*Farquhar* et al., 1982].

The Philippine mass media campaign was also based on the concepts of persuasive communication. However, in contrast to the Three-Community Study it used radio only as the mass medium of communication and was designed to encourage the *addition* of calorie- and protein-dense foods and a source of vitamin A – specifically fish, oil and green vegetables – to the weaning food (rice gruel) of infants. The campaign was evaluated by means of surveys assessing changes in knowledge, attitude and behavior. Rates of actual adoption of the supplement and the decision-making process were both measured. Statistically significant numbers of mothers adopted the recommendations of the messages, and their changed behavior was accompanied by large-scale shifts in attitude and knowledge. Although the project was designed to test the effectiveness of radio alone, extension workers who heard the messages incorporated them into their own teaching, and as was true in the Stanford study, such face-to-face education along with the radio messages was more effective in producing change than either educational intervention alone [*Zeitlin and Formacion,* 1981]. Other mass media projects have not been as thoroughly evaluated as the ones described here but they are usually reported as having had some positive effects by whatever the criteria used [*Leslie,* 1977]. It should be noted that although the mass media campaigns described were large-scale and involved highly skilled professionals from many disciplines, the messages were based on the needs of the intended learners as assessed locally or derived from national health statistics.

B. Community Programs

Growth in mass media use during the past decade has been complemented by a trend toward community-based programs in which local people together with extension workers and other health professionals provide nutrition education and related services to others in their communities [*Zeitlin and Formacion,* 1981]. These non-formal, community-level interventions have been carried out on a group or one-to-one basis in a variety of settings, such as senior citizen centers, food assistance programs, hospitals, health centers and workplace cafeterias. *Zeitlin* [1977] notes that in developing countries face-to-face non-formal nutrition educational activities are usually offered in conjunction with health services.

This observation calls attention to one of the important changes that has taken place in the content – as distinguished from the methods – of what is thought of as nutrition education in recent years. In a 1977 review for the USAID, *Rasmuson* noted that during the previous decade there had been a great expansion in the subjects that were viewed as 'proper concerns' for nutrition education in developing countries, and that nutrition education now included much more than 'merely counseling people on the basic food groups and how to prepare meals'. Nutrition education was now seen to include all those factors which affect the 'flow of food nutrients from the farm to utilization by the consumer' [*Rasmuson,* 1977].

Education in nutrition may now include instruction and/or demonstration on such food production topics as the increased cultivation of fruits, vegetables and legumes, the raising and dressing of small animals, improved fertilization and cropping practices, improved food storage practices, and so on. Nutrition education is also recognized as appropriately encompassing a whole range of 'health' topics which impact on nutrition by affecting the learner's nutrient needs: the causes and signs of disease, the value of immunization, the importance of sanitation and so on, since such interventions which prevent nutrient 'leakage' have a major impact on nutritional status. Moreover, appropriate dietary topics are no longer limited to such traditional ones as teaching proper diets and appropriate weaning foods to pregnant and nursing women, but may include information on dangers associated with bottle-feeding or with certain intra-family food distribution practices.

It is worth noting that similar 'non-nutritional' interventions at the community level are also being recognized as part of the nutrition educator's appropriate concern in developed countries. Urban vegetable gardening has expanded enormously in many countries both as a method of organizing poor urban neighborhoods and as a way of helping increase vegetable consumption among the poor.

Such a broadened focus seems to grow naturally out of the fact that the strategies used in non-formal community-based programs are often derived from the self-actualizing school of educational psychology described earlier, in which the time, place, and manner of instruction are learner-centered.

Clearly such strategies do not allow for a restrictive definition of either how or by whom identified nutritional problems are to be solved.

Teaching strategies in community programs often involve the use of growth charts when dealing with mothers of infants, and the use of stories, games, projective picture stories, oral tradition and drama, as well as various visual aids such as posters, calendars or comic books. Such consciousness raising or informational adjuncts are often combined with skill training – i.e. people are provided with the opportunity to practice, with guidance and corrective feedback, behaviors they have learned through instruction or modeling. These approaches and others in non-formal education are described in detail by *Srinavasan* [1977] and *Zeitlin and Formacion* [1981]. In sum, the experiences of the past decade confirm the conclusion *Whitehead* reached in 1970 – that active participation by learners in the design and implementation of nutrition education is a distinguishing characteristic of programs that are successful in improving nutritional practice. The degree of participation of the learners in the various phases of the process depends of course on the specific project involvement.

In Project Poshak, for example, nutrition education complemented a large supplemental feeding program for preschool children and pregnant and lactating mothers involving 500 villages in 12 districts in India. Nutrition education was conducted in the homes of beneficiaries and their families – since this was the final delivery point for the food – but the medical staff of the health centers and satellite subcenters actually did the educating [Clearinghouse, 1982]. On the other hand, in a project in the Philippines designed to improve the nutritional status of resettled squatters, interested local women were trained in various nutritionally healthful practices and these 'nutrition instructors' then taught what they had learned to 3–5 families in their homes [*Bartolome,* 1977]. Finally, in a Save the Children Federation project in Mexico [*Terreri,* 1977] an SCF staff member, along with a local social workers, visited every home in ten communities and talked with the women about community needs. Program plans were then based on problems and solutions decided upon at group meetings attended by the women. In this way, the problems identified and the solutions offered were appropriate (and different) for each of the communities, and local women were involved in all stages of planning, decision-making and program implementation.

Descriptions of many other projects can be found elsewhere [INCS; Clearinghouse, 1982; *Shack,* 1977]. Clearly, face-to-face non-formal nutrition education complements the use of mass media. Face-to-face contact is, on the whole, considered more effective; mass media can reach more people more quickly. A combination of both would, of course, represent the best strategy. To assist countries in their efforts to use both, the International Nutrition Communication Service [*Nestor* et al., in press] is assembling a comprehensive catalogue of materials for use in mass media and face-to-face nutrition education in developing countries.

VIII. Formal Nutrition Education

Since schooling is near universal in the developed countries and increasingly so – at least at the elementary school level – in developing countries, nutrition education in the schools has usually been considered a potentially important means of teaching a large proportion of the world's population. About 81% of the children in Latin America, 68% in Asia, and 40% in Africa attend primary schools [United Nations, 1981]. However, most children attend for no more than 4 or 5 years and the yearly dropout rates from first grade on may be 50% or even more. Secondary schools have a much smaller enrollment than primary schools and tend to serve the more affluent populations in the cities.

Not all children are in school, however, and not all countries provide nutrition education to those who are. In 1976, UNESCO conducted a comprehensive survey of 135 countries to learn the status of nutrition education in educational systems [*Calloway* et al., 1979]. 39% of the 69 countries that responded indicated that they included nutrition education in the pre-primary grades; 71% included it in the primary grades and 74% in the secondary grades. Encouraging as these figures seem, they do not really inform us about the actual extent of nutrition education throughout a given country. For example, the USA was one of the countries answering that there was nutrition education at pre-school, primary and secondary levels. Yet in a comprehensive study done at about the same time, only 30% of US state education agencies and 40% of local school districts reported that they had any programs or projects in nutrition education [Education Commission, 1975].

There are a number of reasons why the implementation of nutrition education may have been so spotty despite the apparent ready availability of a captive audience. Among them are the following: First, most school curricula are already crowded with many subjects generally viewed as of greater importance than nutrition. 'Lack of time' was listed as one of the major blocks to implementation in the UNESCO survey. A second problem mentioned in the survey was lack of qualified personnel. While high schools have specialists who may be able to teach some nutrition – e.g. science and home science/home economics teachers – elementary school teachers are generalists whose preparation has not usually included specific training in nutrition.

Third, during the past decades, much of nutrition education that has been implemented in schools has been based more on the needs of the field than on the needs of the learners; i.e. it has tended to emphasize the principles of nutrition science as its content. In a 1976 analysis of major curriculum guides used in the USA, *Cooper and Go* [1976] found that the objectives of the teaching units were primarily in the cognitive domain with most requiring only knowledge and comprehension of nutrition information. And in a 1980 review of elementary school studies, programs and curricula in the USA, *Contento* found an emphasis on nutrients and the Basic Four Food Groups system [*Contento,* 1981]. Only a minority of the curricula emphasized issues that probably ought to be of concern in a developed country – how to avoid excessive amounts of fat, sugar and salt in the diet and how to choose among the many foods that do not fit easily into the four food groups. In the UNESCO survey too, 'research findings' topped the list of resources 'found useful in drawing up a relevant curriculum in nutrition education' [*Calloway* et al., 1979], a clear indication of an emphasis on nutrition science.

Fourth, although *Whitehead* concluded that the most successful approaches to improving food habits were those which emphasized the active participation of the learner, *Cooper and Go* [1976] found that the curriculum guides in use in the USA in 1976 were quite teacher dominated, did not provide for active participation of students, and suggested evaluation procedures that were mostly tests of knowledge with the recall of information predominating [*Cooper and Go,* 1976]. The UNESCO survey, too, found that 'lecture' was the most often utilized method of instruction, being used 'frequently' by 50% of the countries. Demonstrations and discussions were used 'frequently' by 39 and 32% of the countries, respectively. However, the method most often listed as one they would like to develop further was education through 'demonstration', followed by 'practice by students' and 'small group work'. Use of audiovisuals, the discovery method, and debates were other strategies suggested by a few respondents. The barriers to implementing these desired methods were given as 'financial' by 68% of the countries, followed by lack of 'familiarity with methods' (41%) and lack of 'familiarity with aids' (31%).

These problems are of course interrelated. When nutrition education is viewed as lecturing about nutrition science, most elementary – and even high school – teachers do not consider teaching this subject as pressing as other educational needs. Nor do they consider themselves as qualified to teach it. Clearly, if nutrition education is to receive wider endorsement by teachers, nutrition education in the school setting must break out of this cycle.

To solve the first problem – lack of time – nutrition can be integrated into existing curricula. The FAO notes [FAO, 1971] that although the two approaches – teaching nutrition as a separate subject area in the elementary schools, or introducing nutrition messages into subject areas already taught – have not been 'properly compared by simultaneous evaluation in similar groups, it would seem a priori, that an uninterrupted educatory process, well developed, would be preferable to a separate subject'.

Furthermore, we argued earlier that nutrition science was an insufficient basis for nutrition education and that the relevance of the content to the learner's needs had to be taken into account. We note here that a change in the nature of the content, accompanied by appropriate new curricula and aids may also increase the relevance of nutrition education from the teacher's standpoint as well as increasing teacher's perceptions of their own competence to teach the subject – thus contributing to the solution of the other problems raised above.

In the USA, these issues have begun to be seriously addressed within the last 5 years. One of the stimuli for what has been a sudden burst of activity was a 1977 act of Congress which established the Nutrition Education and Training Program (NETP) providing money for school nutrition education in every state. The NETP legislation specifically directed schools to integrate nutrition education in the classroom with the serving of school meals and, in many states, funding was provided to local school districts on the basis of competitive proposals for innovative nutrition education. One result has been a reconceptualization of both the content and the methods of nutrition education.

Thus, as in non-formal settings, the content of school nutrition education in the USA has begun to address more adequately the nutrition related problems of today's affluent societies, problems such as heart disease, diabetes, cancer and hypertension. Many of the newly developed curricula go beyond the presentation of information on the traditional food groups and nutrients. Instead, the admonitions of the Dietary Guidelines – to eat more fiber, complex carbohydrates, fruits and vegetables, and to eat less sugar, fat, and salt – are often made primary. In addition, the curricula attempt to help children develop the knowledge and skills needed to choose intelligently from among large numbers of unequally nutritious foods as well as to evaluate dietary advice which comes sought and unsought from unequally reliable sources. Many aspects of food are discussed in these curricula – not just their nutrient content – and the social, cultural, economic and environmental contexts of food behavior are often examined.

The new programs and curricula have also become more learner-centered in their methods. A comprehensive review of nutrition education in 1980 conducted for the NET Program indicated that many of the curricula had by then come to emphasize the active participation of students in the learning process [*Nestor and Glotzer,* 1981]. A review of curricula designed even more recently confirms this trend [Nutrition Education Resources Project, 1982]. The presentation formats of these curricula are lively and topics are covered in a way that is relevant to the lives of today's children and adolescents. The importance of exercise is also often emphasized. Most of the curricula are designed to integrate food and nutrition education with the teaching of other subjects.

The UNESCO survey suggests that in the developing countries too the needs of the learner are increasingly used to shape formal nutrition education. Thus although research findings topped the list of sources important for curriculum development, other sources, in descending order of importance, were: past experience with nutrition education; reports on social and cultural problems; special inquiry on needs of population, and economic reports. In addition the survey indicates that in some parts of the world nutrition education has been integrated with school feeding programs much the way the NET Program in the USA has made an effort to link lunchroom and schoolroom.

In response to the needs revealed in its own survey and at the 1977 nutrition education conference sponsored by UNESCO and IUNS [*Sinclair and Howat,* 1980], UNESCO has now produced a document designed to assist primary school teachers in the task of integrating nutrition education in the curriculum [UNESCO, 1981]. It consists of lesson units contributed as examples by teachers from all over the world.

While there is evidence that food habits that develop during childhood and adolescence are important in determining adult eating patterns, the school is, of course, only one source of influence on these patterns. Given the limitations on what the school can achieve, *Bartels* [1980] and others have urged that what goes on in the school should complement, reinforce, and be reinforced by non-formal education within the community, as well as by such other sources of influence on dietary practices as health care facilities, economic resources and access to food.

IX. Evaluation of Nutrition Education Programs

Over the years a number of observers have commented on the lack of evaluation in both formal and non-formal nutrition education efforts [e.g. *Bagchi,* 1977; *McNaughton,* 1977; *McKenzie and Mumford,* 1965; *White,* 1973]. And yet evaluation is crucial to nutrition education. Without it, we cannot determine whether our programs are effective, let alone how to design them to make them more effective.

There are, of course, many obstacles to evaluation, as *Brun* [1981] has noted. Many practitioners do not see the need for structured or quantifiable procedures of evaluation and therefore do not allow time for it. Others are afraid that the evaluation may point to inadequate performance on their part or be misinterpreted in a way that is unfavorable to them. Financial constraints also present a problem. With limited funds or personnel it may be felt that the money is better spent providing the service than evaluating it. Political considerations, too, influence the evaluation process. The survival of many programs – and hence the jobs of nutrition educators – depends on government or other funding sources and, for many in the programs, it may appear better not to evaluate at all than to come up with results that are contrary to the expectations of these funding sources.

Even where there is the willingness, or indeed desire, to evaluate programs, the methodological problems are still formidable. There are no simple instruments that are conveniently available in some kind of sourcebook for the nutrition educator to simply look up and apply to a given population in a given situation. Other dilemmas that have been described by *Green* [1977] for health education apply to nutrition education as well. Rigorously designed evaluations require strict adherence to carefully specified protocols. We may, therefore, end up with results that are scientifically rigorous but trivial or not generalizable to other situations. The timing of the evaluation is also a dilemma since there may be a delay in the impact, or a decay in the impact with time, a backlash from the cessation of the program, or changes in society with time that augment or undermine the effect of the program.

The most important dilemma, however, lies in the fundamental issue of what really are appropriate parameters to evaluate. Where there *has* been evaluation, especially in school programs, it has tended to be based on increases in nutrition knowledge. In the 1976 UNESCO survey, for example, 81% of the countries indicated that the evaluation of nutrition education programs in their schools was based on knowledge [*Calloway* et al., 1979]. *Contento* in her 1980 review of school nutrition education programs in the USA found the same trend [*Contento,* 1981].

Yet as we pointed out earlier, the goal of nutrition education is to improve the well-being of people. Thus improvement in the nutritional status or in the food-related behaviors of the target population would seem to be more appropriate indicators of success than knowledge gains. Unfortunately, as *St. Pierre* [1982] has pointed out, nutritional status outcomes occur only after the passage of time, are generally of small magnitude, and are often difficult to measure. In addition, it is often impossible to prove that new behaviors resulted solely from the educational intervention because so many other environmental factors may have intervened.

On the other hand, those outcomes that are observed immediately at the conclusion of an educational intervention may be large, easily measured, and more readily attributable to the educational intervention, but – unfortunately – relationships between these outcomes and nutritional well-being are indirect, complex and unclear. Examples of such outcomes would be gains in knowledge or more favorable attitudes toward nutrition as assessed by some sort of attitude survey.

The dilemma of which of these parameters to use is well exemplified by comparing two sets of comments. *Bagchi* [1980], in describing the evaluation experience of the Applied Nutrition Programme, sponsored by UNICEF in collaboration with the FAO and WHO, said: 'When it came to the question of evaluating the nutrition education component, the matter had to be dropped since no suitable parameters were identified. There was reluctance, quite justifiably, to use health parameters like height and weight of the child population' [*Bagchi,* 1980]. Congressman *Richmond* of the USA, on the other hand, stated: 'The old numbers game of counting prints that leave the shelves, and faces encountered in meeting rooms is pointless. If the Congress is to provide the dollars and the policy initiatives to fuel a national nutrition education program, we must be assured that it will accomplish significant improvement in the health and well-being of citizens' [*Richmond,* 1977].

Nutrition educators in the USA have attempted to take this charge seriously in the past 5 years. Thus the NET Program evaluation was based not only on increases in nutrition knowledge, and changes in reported food preferences and food-related attitudes, but also on the amount of food wasted at school meals and other behavioral measures [*St. Pierre and Rezmovic,* 1982]. The Five-City Project has also carefully stipulated that it aims to bring about 'a 10% reduction in overall cardiovascular risk status in 2 years' [*Farquhar* et al., 1982]. Curricula designed for schools are also now routinely evaluated for their impact on behavior as well as on knowledge and attitudes [see *St. Pierre and Rezmovic,* 1982; *Brun,* 1981; *Shannon* et al., 1981]. And recently, the Journal of Nutrition Education (JNE) devoted an entire issue to measurement and evaluation instruments that have been used in nutrition education [JNE, 1981].

However, many conceptual and methodological issues remain. There is still some controversy over the extent to which nutrition educators should be accountable for behavior change in the target population. *St. Pierre* [1982] notes that policy makers and program practitioners often have different opinions regarding appropriate indicators of effectiveness and that a fair evaluation must take into account the differing needs of the various groups involved. This theme is echoed in *Zeitlin's* [1977] evaluation model. She suggests that the parameters of nutrition knowledge, attitudes, behavior, and nutritional status indicators should all be measured, if possible. Such measurements can be viewed as complementary, and each parameter can assist in the interpretation of the others. However, such an approach does not resolve the issue of which variable to use to judge program effectiveness. For example, the mass media campaign in the Philippines [*Cooke and Romweber,* 1977] resulted in significant increases in mothers' knowledge about and favorable attitudes towards adding oil to their infants' weaning food – rice gruel. It even resulted in significant increases in the number of mothers who actually put oil in their infants' weaning food (i.e. changed behavior in the intended direction). But the amount of oil added was not sufficient to improve significantly the infants' weights. Which results should be used to judge the program's success?

These and many other issues in evaluation have received considerable attention in the past 5 years and have given rise to the emerging field of evaluation research in nutrition education [see for example *Wolf,* 1977; *Brun,* 1980a, b; *Talmadge* et al., 1978; *Sims and Light,* 1980; *Kolbe,* 1979; *Ward,* 1981; *Zeitlin and Formacion,* 1981].

X. Informal Nutrition Education

Intentional education, it has long been observed, is carried out not only by those officially designated educators; other institutions in society also have systematic curricula which they teach quite deliberately over time [see e.g. *Potter,* 1958]. Among these are families, businesses, religions, libraries, day-care centers, newspapers and magazines and radio and television stations. We will consider here only the latter. Their curricula include not only 'programs labeled educational, but also news broadcasts and documentaries (which presumably inform), commercials (which teach people to want) and soap operas (which reinforce common myths and values)' [*Cremin,* 1975].

That *all* of these media messages educate is a cause of concern since the media in many developing countries are not under the control of those promoting public welfare. *Fuglesang* [1975] once observed that African air waves were very largely taken up by programs from 'international information monopolies' and that 'the system functions like a vacuum cleaner which sucks up whatever software is strategically placed in its vicinity'. It does not require such imagination to be concerned over the impact on a poor country of the values conveyed by many of the most popular (and hence most widely exported) programs. A recent and much-attacked report on media relationships between the developed and developing worlds has raised a number of important 'educational' questions regarding these and other exports [*McBride,* 1980].

One educational input from the mass media has been particularly attacked in both developed and developing countries as having had a detrimental effect on eating habits – namely the food product advertising which the media disseminate. The educational goal of advertisements for consumable substances is to teach people to want certain products and/or the social life which their promotion associates with consuming those products. There is an increasing body of evidence showing that this education may be having at least some negative nutritional effects, especially among children even though research has not been able to address the effects of long-term cumulative exposure to advertising [see e.g. *Adler* et al., 1980]. In the developing world, most attention has been focused on whether infant formula promotion to poor and illiterate mothers has contributed to a decline in breast-feeding and a consequent increase in infant malnutrition [e.g. *Greiner,* 1975; *Groener,* 1980; *Hamilton,* 1982; IUNS, 1982; *Jelliffe,* 1972; *Pelto,* 1981a, b; UNICEF, 1982]. However, the 'bottle babies' controversy is simply a highly visible example of how activities designed to sell products may serve to promote or accelerate value transfer in ways unintended by (and objectionable to) official educating agencies.

Although there is a great disparity between the amounts invested in advertising in poor and rich countries, almost everywhere the total invested in advertising food and drink will exceed the funds available for official nutrition education and other health promotion activities. As the poor learn to be consumers – so critics contend – they seek to become part of the modern world by using up their limited resources on such of its symbols as they can afford – e.g. soft drinks and snack foods [see e.g. *Barnett and Muller,* 1974].

That people learn from everything around them is obvious; indeed, as we observed in discussing the origins of nutrition education, culture took care of teaching about good eating through most of human history. So the problem is not that children come to classrooms or mothers to nutrition centers as persons already implanted with a variety of cultural messages about food. They always did. What is new is the increase in the number of those messages that are commercial. Because commercial messages are not designed to teach people how to purchase the best diet possible at the lowest coast, but to sell products, they can create a distorted image of which products are essential, desirable and cheap. Among the affluent, such distortion may merely contribute to an excess of obesity and cavities; but mistakes in food purchasing in populations where there is less margin for financial or nutritional risk may have much more serious health repercussions.

In this regard, another trend reported in the UNESCO survey of formal nutrition education is disturbing in that it suggests that product promotion may not cease at the door of the classroom [*Calloway* et al., 1979]. 48% of the respondents indicated that they found food industry printed matter from within their countries to be a useful teaching resource in the classroom; 32% said they used such materials from another country. An extensive review of such materials several years ago concluded that they were of varying quality, were sometimes intentionally misleading or blatantly promotional, and were almost always a problem educationally in that they emphasized processed products which it was profitable to promote [*Gussow,* 1979]. Appropriate nutritional messages for the poor – as we have reiterated – are likely to be lessons on what to add to the diet to increase its nutritional value, but 'the foods that most need adding are not the comparatively expensive processed products from which the food industry profits most (but) simple, locally available foods' whose promotion it would be difficult for processors to afford [*Gussow,* 1979]. *Gussow* concluded that it was especially 'important for countries where advertising and promotion are ostensibly targeted at an affluent minority to ensure that promotional materials are kept out of both formal and informal systems of education designed for the poor' [*Gussow,* 1979].

XI. Nutrition Education: Who Is Ignorant?

The controversy over product promotion, especially the promotion of infant formula, has contributed to a much more fundamental dialogue about the role of educators where hunger is involved. Before the USA cast the lone dissenting vote on the Infant Formula Marketing Code, formula manufacturers spent a good deal of time in Washington 'educating' US policy makers. Advocates in turn spent a good deal of time in Geneva 'educating' colleagues at the working sessions which produced the marketing code. Would the efforts of nutrition educators in certain circumstances be better directed toward policy makers than toward the poor? *Bartels* [1980], commenting on the UNESCO survey of nutrition education efforts around the world, comments that the North West Europeans considered 'the existence of a national nutrition policy would be more effective (than education) in improving nutrition and that changes in economic status influence eating habits at a much faster rate than education' [*Bartels,* 1977]. Although the issue of national food policies or of national control over food marketing activities is well beyond the scope of this review, it should be observed that such options exist and that nutrition educators may well feel that implementing the Infant Formula Marketing code in their own countries so as to help prevent miseducation of mothers is a priority activity. That policy-making is not the whole answer, however, is suggested by the fact that Norway's model nutrition policy has not yet had the hoped-for impact on food consumption [*Ringen,* 1983].

Nonetheless, the suggestion that policy may be more effective than education raises the issue of who it is that needs to be educated – and about what – when a country suffers from widespread hunger and malnutrition. Is the nutrition educator obliged to worry about the learner having *enough* to eat? What is the role of nutrition education if people do not have food? *Zeitlin and Formacion* [1981] define nutrition education as 'any communications system that teaches people to make better use of available food resources', thus suggesting that increasing the resources to be made use of is probably someone else's task. But *Longacre* [1978] has captured the dilemma that actually confronts the nutrition educator in the field. 'The basic hypothesis of most nutrition education is that improved nutritional standards would be achieved if people made better use of the resources already available. Behavioral change is expected from the malnourished persons themselves – or their parents. But sooner or later, every honest nutritionist working in a poverty situation faces moments of truth in which the solutions are perceived to lie elsewhere.'

Such dilemmas are not limited to poor countries. In the USA nutrition aides, trained under the well-funded EFNEP program to help the poor improve their food selection skills, find it difficult to concentrate on teaching the four food groups to a family whose refrigerator is empty or, worse, out on the street because an eviction has occurred [*Rifkind,* 1982]. Yet it is clear that much of what we call nutrition education has not only failed to address these problems but has to a very large extent not even acknowledged them as part of professional concern.

Almost a decade ago *Berg* [1976] commented on the non-involvement of nutrition professionals in the issue of world hunger, noting that the profession suffered from 'a too narrow perception of appropriate roles and responsibilities'. Pointing to critical decisions to be made in the following decades which would influence nutrition around the world, he commented that 'although contributions from the laboratory and the clinic will continue to be important, their significance in terms of the nutritional status of the population may well be overshadowed by forces and institutions that heretofore were in no way regarded as part of the nutritionist's domain' [*Berg,* 1976]. *Berg's* comments imply that if nutrition educatorss are to meet the needs of all learners, they must develop a wider conception of their task. This role of the nutrition educator, as one who questions 'why certain segments of the population are denied access to the means of adequate nutrition and how such means can be secured for them', was articulated almost simultaneously in two recent documents: one was the report of a 1978 meeting held at Dar es Salaam, Tanzania, by Committee II/10 of the International Union of Nutrition Sciences for the purpose of 'Rethinking Nutrition Education Under Changed Socio-economic Conditions', first published in full in April of 1980 [Rethinking, 1980]; the other was an issue of the *Teachers College Record* entitled 'Learning and Eating: The New Nutrition Education' which was published 1 month later [*Gussow,* 1980b].

Both these documents urged that nutrition educators could no longer confine themselves to their traditional concerns – nutritious foods and balanced diets – and that it was not even enough simply to expand the topics and skills it is acceptable to teach, to include, for example, vegetable gardening and sanitation. In order to be effective, nutrition education would 'have to concern itself not only with what people eat, how they eat it, and how what they eat affects them, but indeed with whether they have anything to eat at all – and if not, why not' [*Gussow,* 1980a].

It is not clear to what extent nutrition educators generally accept this version of their role, although as we pointed out earlier, there appears to be widespread support for the notion that concern with food may include a concern with a good part of the food chain. Attempting to evaluate the impact of their reassessment document, Committee II/10 of IUNS sent copies of the document and an accompanying questionnaire to 1,852 persons, largely readers of the UNU *Food and Nutrition Bulletin,* in April of 1981. Under the headline 'Who is Ignorant?' they asked, among other things, whether the term nutrition education should be restricted to diet, nutrient and health information or broadened and, if broadened, in what manner. Of the 318 persons (18%) who responded to the questionnaire as a whole, 300 answered this question and 92% of these said the term should be broadened. The new elements to be included – in order of preference – were 'sociocultural context' 88%, 'local participation' 86%, 'environmental resource base' 81%, 'patterns of control of resources' 73%, and 'international food policy' 73% [*Eide and Mosio,* 1981].

It is impossible to judge the representativeness of those who responded to the questionnaire (or even received it initially). It is also hard to know just how respondents interpreted the question. Asked to give examples of 'special projects' of their own that might 'provide a satisfactory approach to information about causes of nutritional problems as well as to ways of remedying them', 76% of the respondents listed such projects, but a high percentage of them involved fairly conventional nutrition education activities [*Mosio,* 1982].

It is perhaps more indicative of the increasing acceptance of food availability as a proper concern for nutrition educators that the topic 'Access to Food' was the theme of the 1981 Annual Meeting of the Society for Nutrition Education. In her keynote address to that meeting, *Eide* [1982] noted that the problem of deciding which facts to present (discussed earlier in relation to the goals of nutrition education) arises again when one attempts to explain why some people do and others do not have food. What are 'the *causes* for differences in access to food?' she asked, and answered by pointing out that 'various people have their various models'. Among these are the *Population Explosion Model* ('there are too many mouths to feed, hence there is too little food'), the *Poverty Model* ('people are poor and malnourished due to a lack of resources'), and the *Conflict of Interest Model* ('strong conflicts exist between different interest groups' leading to non-equitable distribution of resources). *Eide* [1982] noted, however, that: 'To have chosen a model for explanation does not automatically lead to understanding what the role of the nutrition educator can or should be [so that] the actual activity in which the nutritionist or nutrition educator becomes involved will often have to be a compromise between the ideal and the possible.'

More recently *Schuftan* [1982] has once again addressed the question of what role nutritionists do and should play in a world they judge unjust. It is not enough, he argues, to be a generalized humanitarian or even a liberal; a conscientious nutritionist must necessarily be ideological, willing to raise much more fundamental political questions especially about 'helping' interventions that are clearly not addressing the real problems of the poor. The problem, as *Schuftan* [1982] points out, is that: 'Certain actions that ... will have a lasting effect and combat malnutrition ... are mostly non-nutritional, at least at the outset.' Nevertheless, he argues: 'Nutritionists have to stop thinking that they cannot contribute much to the selection and implementation of non-nutritional interventions because they are outside our immediate field of expertise.'

Whatever nutrition educators can *do* about the fact, they must acknowledge that so long as acute and chronic undernutrition and suffering exist in a world with enough food for everyone, and so long as propaganda convinces the poor to buy expensive and/or nutritionally impoverished foods and drinks, then nutrition education is palliative at best if it is limited simply to teaching people how best to husband their inadequate resources in the face of temptation. On the other hand, it is also important to acknowledge that merely eliminating inequities in access to food – or advertising – will not assure dietary adequacy.

There is a not-always-articulated assumption among the politically thoughtful that if the poor were only given control over their own resources, they would all be well fed, either because their agricultures and their diets would return to some sort of 'traditional' (and presumably optimal) pattern, or because they would wisely use technology to move forward unerringly toward a well-nourished future. 'I believe this project and all other types of nutrition education in developing countries are only interim solutions ... When incomes reach a level sufficient to feed the family, there will be no need to teach the feeding of protein' [*Drummond,* 1975]. Though the subject is too large to explore here in any depth, it must be pointed out again that there is little to support the notion that good nutrition will automatically be assured by guaranteeing access to money and food. Not all traditional diets were optimal, and there is no evidence that in an environment containing a variety of processed foods wise selections will be made. Just as it is true that without some serious attention to redistribution there is little hope that people will be well fed, it is also true that even if access to food is assured intelligent decisions about which foods to produce and eat will require the help of those trained in nutrition. After all, children living amid an abundance of green leaves now suffer blindness because their parents do not know how they can use those leaves to prevent it.

XII. Nutrition Education and the Needs of Society

We have pointed out earlier that the content of education derives from the needs of a discipline, the needs of learners and the needs of a society. And we have discussed how the first two of these needs might affect nutrition education. The psychological/educational theories we have reviewed and their application in formal and informal nutrition education are clearly efforts at understanding the learner, at determining what kinds of lessons, in what kinds of settings, different kinds of learners can make the best use of. We have also asked, in relation to learners, whether it is appropriate for nutrition educators to take actions aimed at increasing their access to food. What, then, of the needs of society?

Tyler [1950], discussing this aspect of curriculum building, notes that it was an increase in the amount of confirmed information available as a result of science and the industrial revolution, that made it necessary to choose what things schools would teach. With so much knowledge available, schools had to select that which was relevant to contemporary life [*Tyler,* 1950]. Where nutrition education is concerned, the term *relevant* has been very largely equated with the word *practical.* What is relevant in that sense is what will equip persons to make optimal use of the food supply so as to improve or maintain their own health. Even the more radical political analyses aim only at assuring the individual fair access to that food supply. The underlying social goal, however, remains the same – well-fed children and adults, who can be better learners and happier more productive workers. Guaranteeing the good nutrition of individuals has, in short, been viewed as meeting society's needs.

As we near the end of the 20th century, however, it is becoming clearer that the 'needs of society' means something more than simply the nutritional health of individuals. Just as it is not enough to teach wise food selection if there is not enough food to select from; just as teaching gardening, co-oping, hygiene, and other food production and nutrient conservation skills will not improve nutritional status in the absence of resources that will enable learners to utilize their newfound skills [*Ritenbaugh,* 1981; *Schuftan,* 1982]; just so will a sustainable society need individuals capable of thinking beyond their personal survival [*Gussow,* 1980c, 1981a]. In the current crisis of resource availability and environmental stability, distributional injustice is only one of the factors moving the world to the brink of ecological catastrophe [*Eckholm,* 1982]. While there is disagreement about the time frame of the constraints implied by the term 'limits to growth', there is a much greater degree of consensus that humanity's relationship to the natural environment has reached a crisis point in many parts of the world [see e.g. *Holdgate* et al., 1982; State of the Environment, 1982; United States Department of State, 1980]. Indeed, even *Kahn* [1976], the American influential optimist regarding humanity's affluent future, now admits that his optimism is 'guarded', though he insists that only a 'perverse combination of bad luck and bad management' can derail us. However, among the problems of a 'superindustrial world economy' that he acknowledges *good* luck and *good* planning will have to confront are 'ecological catastrophes', 'genetic calamity', 'pandemics', and 'Armageddon' [*Kahn,* 1982]. Thus some concern for sustainability seems appropriate.

One of the most important things we count upon the natural environment to produce for us is food. Unless we sustain our food-producing capacity, both educational and distributional problems will become moot – however, much wisdom and justice may be desired. Thus, where nutrition education is concerned, society's needs now require that we produce persons knowledgeable enough about their food systems to demand that their leaders act to preserve them.

The ecological crisis as it relates to sustainable food-producing systems has been thoroughly reviewed elsewhere [see e.g. *Davis,* 1979; *Eckholm,* 1976; *Gussow,* 1978; *Lappe,* 1982; *Sampson,* 1982]. Here, in a recent summary, is its essence: 'Ecological systems ... provide us with a wide variety of free public services that are essential to industrial society. ... Yet those services most involved in supplying humanity with nourishment – providing food from the sea and supporting agriculture – are already faltering. World per-capita food reserves have dropped back to their record lows of the mid-1970s, and options for dealing with future production shortfalls are becoming fewer while the probability of such shortfalls occurring is rapidly increasing. In the prairies of central North America – the last bastion of large, dependable grain surpluses – there is now no land kept fallow in soil banks. Indeed, in some of the richest agricultural areas there and elsewhere, land is being *removed* from cultivation at a high rate by urbanization. Desertification, and waterlogging and salinization of irrigated lands are deleting more farm fields. Erosion is ... a serious threat to sustained productivity. Diminishing returns from fertilizer applications and the narrowing of the genetic base of crops also threaten the ability of farmers to produce ever more food for ever more people. So does the likelihood of weather more normal (that is more variable) than the highly unusual and favorable conditions that prevailed in the middle of the 20th century. For these and other reasons, the prospects for greatly increasing yields to meet the needs of rapidly growing global population are not bright. Neither are the prospects for opening new land. Most of the world's land suitable for agriculture is already under cultivation. Contrary to popular belief, for example, rich soils do not underlie most jungles. In most cases the loss of ecosystem services that accompanies the clearing of tropical forests is much greater than the small (and usually temporary) benefit from the meager amount of additional food grown' [*Erlich and Erlich,* 1982].

Nutrition educators who have become conscious of these problems have recognized that helping to solve them will require not merely new kinds of *activities* aimed at improving nutritional status, but new kinds of *analyses* aimed at discovering what kinds of things about food and its production food consumers will need to know in order to survive. We concluded earlier that the task of nutrition education was to teach people how to acquire, prepare and consume foods that were *good* to eat, and that it was not enough to define food as *good* simply on the basis of its nutrient content. Which charateristics of foods might make them *good* to eat in the face of the world food and environmental crisis?

We suggested earlier that the needs of society now required consumers capable of thinking beyond their personal survival, of taking into account not only their personal health but the health of other consumers on the planet as well as the health of the planetary systems that sustain all of them. Food guidance for the 1980s, especially among the affluent minority, may thus need to be a counsel of restraint. An assessment of the *good*ness of foods may, for example, need to take into account the demands that the production of such foods – bananas and coffee, for example – put on other people's cropland, or on the world's energy supply. Perhaps the 'caloric content' of the aluminum container for a diet soda – 400 cal – should be considered as important in making food choices as the caloric content of what the can contains – 3 cal – when energy is a limited resource. Perhaps the resources used in producing a ready-to-eat cereal – to separate the constituents of the grain, to toast it, and to add a dozen or so vitamins, minerals and flavorings and package the result in a four-color printed box – should be part of the information the consumer takes into account when purchasing the product. In short, characteristics of the food other than its nutrient content, and even other than its flavor or attractiveness, may become increasingly valid measures of its *good*ness.

One characteristic that has become increasingly recognized as contributing to the *good*ness of a food is the degree to which its production contributes to self-reliance. In the past decade it has become clearer that it is risky for people to depend for their basic food supplies on distant croplands. The global supermarket about which food policy analysts spoke in the 1960s and 1970s seems less appealing in a world where ethnic, religious and political hostilities can shut off shipments of fuel or food or both. Moreover, it is difficult to monitor, at a distance, what is happening to the resource base that produces a community's food. Thus there has been a growing interest in a variety of settings in examining the potential of various regions for greater food self-reliance [e.g. *Burrill and Nolfi,* 1979; *Lappe and Collins,* 1977; *Roberts,* 1982; *Tudge,* 1977].

Recognizing the implications of a relocalized food supply for dietary change, some nutrition educators have begun to think of developing principles of food selection by which diets appropriate for various regions might be designed. *Haughton* [1982] has proposed appropriate criteria – in addition to nutritional adequacy and acceptability – for a local diet. She suggests that foods might be evaluated for their 'efficiency' in terms of nutrients produced per unit of land, water, energy, and so on, and urges that the data necessary to make such calculations be generated so that nutrition educators can use it to begin to assemble regionally appropriate food guides [*Haughton,* 1982].

By such criteria, different foods would be defined as 'good' in different places and at different seasons, depending at least in part on their ability to be produced in a manner compatible with ecosystem stability. It is interesting to note that a trend toward giving increasing attention to indigenous foods – and food production systems – was evident in some of the responses to the IUNS survey. A few of the respondents reported on projects devoted to recording, reviving, or retaining indigenous foods, traditional knowledge about wild foods, and traditional methods of food production and preservation. In a time when the ability to produce food in 'austere' circumstances may be invaluable to the survival of the human race, nutrition educators are beginning to operate on the recognition that it is inappropriate to encourage 'white man's food' for people like the Australian aborigines, Amerinds, or Amazonian Indians whose tribal patterns of food procurement and production enabled them to thrive in a variety of difficult environments [*Kuhlein and Calloway,* 1977].

Thus, for example, a Meals for Millions project on the Papago Indian Reservation in southwest Arizona, USA, is attempting to revive the cultivation of traditional crops and the use of traditional wild foods to help the Indians move back toward food independence [*Anson,* 1981]. *Roddy* [1978] introduced a nutrition education program in Micronesia that encouraged the use of indigenous foods in place of 'expensive and nonessential imported' ones, and *Tudge* [1980] has written a cookbook designed to show how a food self-sufficient England might eat both healthfully and deliciously. *Kuhlein and Calloway* [1977], noting the decline in the use of traditional foods in Hopiland in the US southwest, note that 'funds and encouragement for the agriculture of their traditional food crops would provide considerably more benefits for the Hopi than many of the food programs which have been offered'.

Relocalizing diets would, of course, work against the growing dietary homogeneity which the presence of a global supermarket and the presence of transnational food corporations has encouraged. Regional food patterns based on ecological and nutritional rationality may offer more effective resistance to such homogeneity than have regional food patterns based on tradition alone.

Relocalizing diets would also localize nutrition education, a consequence that might well solve certain problems – especially in countries where educational resources are already overstressed. It is becoming clear that basic literacy among many of the people most in need of education – and food – must be achieved in the native language if it is to be achieved at all [*Dutcher,* 1982]. Yet, many educational materials are published in major languages where there is a sufficiently literate market to make us of them – so as to have the widest possible sale. It is quite unlikely that there will never be nutrition texts, audiovisual aids, or teaching materials in the varieties of languages which are *not* spoken by the world's affluent. But such materials are of less importance in learning about local food production and local food consumption practices. Moreover, teachers and students who participate in the production of locally relevant materials are more likely to become aware of locally urgent food-supply, food-production issues, hence materials so produced are much more likely to influence nutritional status than are teaching materials produced by either educators or food companies based many hundreds or (more likely) many thousands of miles from the site of the lesson. The efforts of local teachers can thus be directed not toward handing out information about nutrition – which, as we have seen, they often feel they do not have – but to helping people learn which questions they need to ask in order to assure themselves an adequate diet now and in the future.

XIII. Trends and Portents

We opened this review by pointing out that the subject of nutrition education was so broad as to defy easy delimitation. We wish to conclude, therefore by noting, if only in passing, several trends which seem very likely to alter humanity's relationship to its food supply in the remainder of the century and hence to alter the role of nutrition educators. These are: (1) urbanization; (2) the wider distribution of 'modern' processed foods, and (3) the growing women's movement.

Given the definition with which we began, that nutrition education is a replacement for cultural wisdom about what is good to eat, it is clear that one of the major environmental changes of the last – and the coming – decades is the rapid displacement or departure of people from settings in which their traditional wisdom about food was functional. Accelerating urbanization, among other things, turns people from knowledgeable food producers into innocent food purchasers. It thus has massive implications for nutrition educators, some of which have been previously noted in this series [*Den Hartog,* 1981].

The growing urban population will be confronted with a steadily increasing number of unfamiliar processed foods whose relative nutritional worth will be difficult for these new consumers to evaluate. The loss of usefulness of craft skills of which we earlier spoke will present even more formidable problems for nutrition educators in developing countries than it has for nutrition educators in the USA, the country which appears to have gone furthest in the direction of novelty in its food supply. One obvious 'solution' that is certain to be proposed – as it has been in the USA – is fortification of the new food products so as to guarantee consumers' dietary adequacy. Except in a very tightly controlled food supply, fortification may well prove (as it has in the USA) to be of highly questionable benefit, and since it tends to destroy natural relationships between certain food classes and certain nutrients (e.g. cornflakes in the USA are now a better source of B_{12} than of thiamine) it may seriously complicate the job of the nutrition educator.

Nutrition education seems, as yet, hardly to have been touched by the women's movement, though the profession is predominantly a female one. That this situation is unlikely to persist is suggested by the increasing attention being given to the role of women in development – and hence in food policy [see e.g. *Boserup,* 1970; *Beneria and Sen,* 1981; *Dauber and Cain,* 1980; FAO, 1979; *Lewis,* undated; *Rogers,* 1980; UNDP, 1980].[6] Commenting on the various UN conferences that preceded the International Women's Year, *Boulding* [1976] commented that 'at each conference it became increasingly clear that the failure of male professionals, administrators and planners to recognize the most elementary facts about women's part in the entire complex of productive processes from child-bearing to agriculture to industry and back to feeding families was leading to disastrous planning and policy errors. Since no technical aid programs were being directed at women, half of the human race stood outside the entire so-called development process' [*Boulding,* 1976].

Some of these same issues have begun to surface in the USA, as part of what is called the New Home Economics [see e.g. *Burns,* 1975; *Evenson,* 1981]. The fact is that women are not merely populations with special nutritional needs but producers of good nutrition and – to an extent too-little recognized – the actual producers of the family food supply in many parts of the world. This means that nutrition educators who are finding themselves increasingly (and necessarily) concerned with 'non-nutritional' issues in a variety of areas will need to add to their concerns the issues of women's status in the family and the community, and the enhancement of women's productive efficiency and access to producer resources. Clearly there is much left to do.

[6] See the publications of International Women's Tribune Center, Inc. (305 East 46th Street, New York, N.Y.); Equity Policy Center (1525 18th Street, N.W., Washington, D.C.); Clearinghouse on Infant Feeding and Maternal Nutrition (1015 15th Street, N.W., Washington, D.C.).

References

Abrahamsson, L.; Velarde, N.: Food classification system for developing countries; in Shack, Teaching nutrition in developing countries or the joys of eating dark green leaves, pp. 113–123 (Meals for Millions, Santa Monica, Calif. 1977).

Adler, R.P.; Lesser, G.S.; Ward, S.: The effects of television advertising on children: review and recommendations (Heath, Lexington 1980).

Ahlström, A.; Räsanen, L.: Review of food grouping systems in nutrition education. J. Nutr. Educ. *5:* 13–17 (1973).

Ajzen, I.; Fishbein, M.: Understanding attitudes and predicting social behavior (Prentice-Hall, Englewood Cliffs 1980).

Anson, C.: The Papago Indian project. Talk at the Society for Nutrition Education Annual Meeting, 1981.

Auerswald, W.; Gergely, S.M. (eds.): Ernährungswissenschaft und Öffentlichkeit (Nutritional Science and the Public). Probleme der Ernährungs- und Lebensmittelwissenschaft, No. 7, p. 25 (1981).

Austin, J.E.; Mahin, M.; Pyle, D.; Zeitlin, M.: Annotated directory of nutrition programs (Harvard Institute for International Development, Cambridge 1978).

Bagchi, K.: Nutrition education through health care systems (WHO); in Sinclair, Howat, World nutrition and nutrition education, pp. 173–185 (Oxford University Press, Oxford 1980).

Baghurst, K.I.; McMichael, A.J.; Record, S.J.; Auricht, C.O.: Interrelationships between dietary intake, dietary knowledge and coronary heart disease risk factors in a group of undergraduate students. Food Nutr. Notes Rev. *37:* 146–151 (1980).

Bandura, A.: Social learning theory (Prentice-Hall, Englewood Cliffs 1977).

Bartels, F.L.: Observations on the UNESCO report on the survey of the position of nutrition within the educational system; in Sinclair, Howat, World nutrition and nutrition education, pp. 137–155 (Oxford University Press, Oxford 1980).

Bartolome, O.C.: Integrated health programs/community aide training; in Shack, Teaching nutrition in developing countries or, the joys of eating dark green leaves (Meals for Millions Foundation, Santa Monica 1977).

Becker, M.H. (ed.): The health belief model and personal health behavior (Slack, Thorofare 1974).

Bell, A.C.; Stewart, A.M.; Radford, A.J.; Cairney, P.T.: A method for describing food beliefs which may predict personal food choice. J. Nutr. Educ. *13:* 22–26 (1981).

Beneria, L.; Sen, G.: Accumulation, reproduction and women's role in economic development: Boserup revisited. Signs *7:* 279–298 (1981).

Berg, A.: Fear of trying. J. Am. diet. Ass. *68:* 311–315 (1976).

Birch, L.L.: Experiential determinants of children's food experiences. Curr. Top. early Childh. Educ. *3:* 29–46 (1980).

Boserup, E.: Woman's role in economic development (Allen & Unwin, London/St. Martins Press, New York 1970).

Bosley, B.: Nutritionists and dietitians in the seventies: trends in education. Wld Rev. Nutr. Diet., vol. 20, pp. 49–65 (Karger, Basel 1975).

Boulding, E.: The underside of history: a view of women through time (Westview Press, Boulder 1976).

Briggs, G.M.: Nutrition education and the food labels. Food Nutr. News *44:* 1, 4 (1973).

Brun, J.: Evaluation of nutrition education: a review; in Nestor, Glotzer, Teaching nutrition, pp. 18–54 (Abt Books, Cambridge 1981).

Brun, J.K. (ed.): Nutrition education research: directions for the future (National Dairy Council, Rosemont 1980a).

Brun, J.K. (ed.): Nutrition education research: strategies for theory-building. Conf. Proc. (National Dairy Council, Rosemont 1980b).

Burns, S.: Home, Inc. (Doubleday & Company, Garden City 1975).

Burrill, G.; Nolfi, J.R.: Strategies for bioregional food systems (Center for Studies in Food Self-Sufficiency, Burlington 1979).

Calloway, D.H.; Gordon, H.F.; Grodner, M.; Pye, O.: Positions of nutrition education within educational systems. ED-77/WS/87 rev. (UNESCO, Paris 1979).

Clark, N.: Tracing the learning approach. World Education Reports, pp. 5–7 (September 1979).

Clearinghouse on Development Communication. Project Profiles. AID studies in educational technology and development communications (USAID Office of Educational Bureau for Science and Technology, Washington 1982).

Coates, T.J.: Eating – a psychological dilemma. J. Nutr. Educ. *13:* suppl., pp. 34–48 (1981).

Commonwealth Department of Health: Report of the National Nutrition Education Conf. (Commonwealth Department of Health, Canberra 1981).

Contento, I.: Kindergarten through sixth grade nutrition education; in Nestor, Glotzer, Teaching nutrition, a review of programs and research (Abt Books, Cambridge 1981).

Contento, I.: Towards a framework for theory-building in nutrition education research; in Brun, Nutrition education research – strategies for theory-building. Conf. Proc. (National Dairy Council, Rosemont 1983).

Cooke, T.M.; Romweber, S.T.: Radio, advertising techniques, and nutrition education: a summary of a field experiment in the Philippines and Nicaragua. Final Report AID Office of Nutrition Contract AID/ta-C-1133 (Manoff International, Washington 1977).

Cooper, D.A.; Go, C.E.: Analysis of nutrition curriculum guides. J. Nutr. Educ. *8:* 62–66 (1976).

Council for Agricultural Science and Technology. Significant issues in nutrition CAST, Ames 1976).

Cremin, L.: Public education and the education of the public. Teach. College Rec. *77:* 1–12 (1975).

Davidson, S.; Passmore, R.; Brock, J.F.; Truswell, A.S.: Human nutrition and dietetics (Churchill-Livingstone, Edinburgh 1979).

Davis, C.: Self-selection of diet by newly weaned infants. Am. J. Dis. Child. *36:* 651–679 (1928).

Davis, C.: Studies in self-selection of diet by young children. J. Am. diet. Ass. *April* (1934).

Davis, C.: Results of the self-selection of diets by young children. Can. med. Ass. J. *41:* 257–261 (1939).

Davis, W.: The seventh year: industrial civilization in transition (Norton, New York 1979).

Dauber, R.; Cain, M.: Women and the technological change in developing countries (Westview Press, Boulder 1980).

Den Hartog, A.: Urbanization, food habits and nutrition. Wld Rev. Nutr. Diet., vol. 38, pp. 112–152 (Karger, Basel 1981).

Dewey, J.: The child and the curriculum (University of Chicago Press, Chicago 1902).

Drummond, T.: Using the method of Paulo Freire in nutrition education: an experimental plan for community action in northeast Brazil. Cornell Int. Nutr. Monogr. Ser. No. 3 (Cornell University Press, Ithaca 1975).

Dutcher, N.: The use of first and second languages in primary education: selected case studies World Bank Staff Working Paper No. 504 (World Bank, Washington 1982).

Dutra de Oliveira, J.E.: Teaching nutrition in medical schools: past, present and future. Wld Rev. Nutr. Diet., vol. 25, pp. 142–165 (Karger, Basel 1976).

Dwyer, J. (ed.): National conference on nutrition education: directions for the 1980s. J. Nutr. Educ. *12:* suppl. 1 (1980).

Eckholm, E.: Losing ground, environmental stress and world food prospects (Norton, New York 1976).

Eckholm, E.: Human wants and misused lands. Natural History *91:* 33–48 (1982).

Education Commission of the States: The status of nutrition education (Education Commission of the States, Denver 1975).

Ehrlich, P.; Erlich, A.: Space age cargo cult. Defenders Wildlife *57:* 2–5 (1982).

Eide, W.B.: The nutrition educator's role in access to food – from individual orientation to social orientation. J. Nutr. Educ. *14:* 15–17 (1982).

Eide, W.; Mosio, M.: Preliminary report from IUNS International Nutrition Education Survey (IUNS Committee II/10, Oslo 1981).

Emergy, M.: The role of the mass media in nutrition education. Commonwealth Department of Health. Report of the National Nutriton Education Conference (Commonwealth Department of Health, Canberra 1981).

Enelow, A.J.; Henderson, A.B. (eds.): Applying behavioral science to cardiovascular risk. Proc. Conf. (Am. Heart Ass., New York 1974).

Evenson, E.: Food policy and the new home economics. Food Policy *6:* 180–193 (1981).

FAO: Joint FAO/WHO Expert Committee on Nutrition. Report on the First Session FAO Nutrition Meetings Report Ser. No. 3 (FAO, Roma 1950).

FAO: Joint FAO/WHO Expert Committee on Nutrition. Fifth Report. FAO Nutrition Meetings Report Ser. No. 19 (FAO, Roma 1958).

FAO: Food and Nutrition education in the primary school. FAO Nutritional Studies No. 25 (FAO, Roma 1971).

FAO: Women in food production, food handling and nutrition. FAO Food and Nutrition Paper, No. 9 (FAO, Roma 1979).

Farquhar, J.W.; Fortmann, S.P.; Jacoby, N.; Haskill, W.L.; Taylor, C.B.; Flora, J.A.; Solomon, D.S.; Rogers, T.; Adler, E.; Breitrose, P.; Weinert, L.: The Stanford five city project: an overview (Stanford Heart Disease Prevention Program/Stanford University, Stanford 1982).

Fidanza, F.; Jelliffe, E.F.P.; Bagchi, K.; Valyasevi, A.; Ju, J.S.; Malatnlema, T.N.; Sarakikya, E.; Cremer, H.D.; Morava, E.; Tarjan, R.; Krehl, W.A.; Taylor, K.B.; Souza, N.; Vannucchi, M.; Dutra de Oliveira, J.E.; Hendrik, A.: Nutrition education and training for health science professionals. Wld Rev. Nutr. Diet., vol. 38, pp. 153–225 (Karger, Basel 1981).

Forbes, A.L.; Pelletier, O.; Keller, W.: Final analysis, 1973–1975 Tunisian national nutrition survey (Tunisian National Institute of Nutrition and Food Technology, Tunis 1979).

Fortmann, S.P.; Williams, P.T.; Hulley, S.B.; Haskell, W.L.; Farquhar, J.W.: Effect of health education on dietary behavior. The Stanford Three Community Study. Am. J. clin. Nutr. *34:* 2030–2038 (1981).

Freire, P.: Pedagogy of the oppressed (Seabury Press, New York 1970).

Friedman, M.P.: Consumer response to unit pricing, open dating and nutrient labeling; in Venkatesan, Proc. 3rd Annu. Conf., pp. 361–369 (Association for Consumer Research, 1972).

Fuglesang, A.: Vested interests and future perspectives in mass communication and media. FAG Bull. *VI:* 13 (1975).

Galst, J.F.; White, M.A.: The unhealthy persuaders: the reinforcing value of television and children's purchase-influencing attempts at the supermarket. Child Dev. *47:* 1089–1096 (1976).

Green, L.W.: Evaluation and measurement: some dilemmas for health education. J. Am. publ. Hlth Ass. *67:* 155–161 (1977).

Greiner, T.: The promotion of bottle feeding by multinational corporations: How advertising and the health professions have contributed. Cornell Int. Nutrition Monogr., No. 2 (Cornell University, Ithaca 1975).

Groener, D.: I'm proud of my industry. Food Monitor *January/February* (1980).

Gussow, J.D.: The feeding web: issues in nutritional ecology (Bull Publishing, Palo Alto 1978).

Gussow, J.D.: Who pays the piper? Food Nutr. *5:* 18–23 (1979).

Gussow, J.D.: Food and nutrition education: a redefinition; in Gussow, Learning and eating: the new nutrition education. Teachers College Rec. *81:* 411–416 (1980a).

Gussow, J.D. (ed.): Learning and eating: the new nutrition education. Teachers College Rec. *81:* 411–525 (1980).

Gussow, J.D.: Nutrition education in a world of limits. Food Nutr. Notes Rev. *37:* 141–145 (1980c).

Gussow, J.D.: Personal food security in the face of impersonal food systems. Ceres *May–June* (1981a).

Gussow, J.D.: Thinking about nutrition education or why is it harder to teach eating than reading? in Wright, Sims, Community nutrition: people, policies and programs (Wadsworth Health Sciences, Monterey 1981b).

Hall, B.L.; Dodds, T.: Voices for development: the Tanzanian national radio study campaigns; in Spanin, Jamison, McAnany, Radio for education and development: case studies, pp. 260–299 (World Bank, Washington 1977).

Hambraeus, I. (ed.): Nutrition in Europe: education, policy and research activities. Proc. 3rd Eur. Nutr. Conf., Upsala 1979 (Almqvist & Wiksell, Stockholm 1980).

Hamilton, L.: Beyond the Nestlé announcement: what the critics say. Food Monitor *May/June* (1982).

Harding, R.: Community nutrition education activities in New South Wales. Commonwealth Department of Health: Report of the National Nutrition Education Conf. (Commonwealth Department of Health, Canberra 1981).

Haughton, B.: The cosmopolitan radish: procedures for constructing a food guide for New York City and State in the Year 2020; unpubl. doct. diss., New York (1982).

Hertzler, A.A.; Anderson, H.L.: Food guides in the United States. J. Am. diet. Ass. *64:* 19–27 (1974).
Hill, M.M.: School lunch – a tool for nutrition education. Wld Rev. Nutr. Diet., vol. 14, pp. 257–268 (Karger, Basel 1972).
Hochbaum, G.M.: Strategies and their rationale for changing people's eating habits. J. Nutr. Educ. *13:* suppl. 1, pp. 59–65 (1981).
Holdgate, M.; White, G.; Kessas, M.: The world environment 1972–82 (United Nations/Tycooly International Press, Dublin 1982).
International Nutrition Communication Service, Education Development Center, Newton, Mass.
Ireton, C.L.; Guthrie, H.A.: Modification of vegetable-eating behavior in preschool children. J. Nutr. Educ. *4:* 100–103 (1972).
IUNS ad hoc task force on rethinking infant nutrition policies and country project teams. Results and policy implications of the cross-national investigation: Rethinking infant nutrition policies under changing socio-economic conditions. Report (1982).
Jacoby, J.; Chestnut, R.W.; Silverman, W.: Consumer use and comprehension of nutrition information. J. Consumer Res. *1977:* 119–128.
Jelliffe, D.B.: Commerciogenic malnutrition. Nutr. Rev. *30:* 199–205 (1972).
Journal of Nutrition Education: Perspectives on nutrition education instrumentation. J. Nutr. Educ. *13:* 83–114 (1981).
Kahn, H.: The next 200 years (Morrow, New York 1976).
Kahn, H.: The coming book (Simon & Schuster, New York 1982).
Kaplowitz, D.C.; Olson, C.M.: The effect of an education program on the decision to breast-feed. J. Nutr. Educ. (in press, 1983).
Karlin, B. (ed.): Summary: the state of the art of delivering low-cost health services in less-developed countries (Am. Public Health Ass., Washington 1977).
Kelman, H.C.: Attitudes are alive and well and gainfully employed in the sphere of action. Am. Psychol. *29:* 310–324 (1974).
Kolasa, K.M.: Nutritional anthropologists and nutrition educators – Potentials for a multidimensional world view. J. Nutr. Educ. *13:* suppl. 1, pp. 9–11 (1981).
Kolbe, L.J.: Evaluating effectiveness – the problems of behavioral criteria. Hlth Educ. *Jan./Feb.:* 12–16 (1979).
Koskela, K.; Puska, P.; Tusmilleto, J.: The North Karelia Project: a first evaluation. Int. J. Hlth Educ. *19:* 59–66 (1976).
Kotler, P.; Zaltman, G.: Social marketing: an approach to planned social change. J. Marketing *35:* 3–12 (1971).
Kuhnlein, H.V.; Calloway, D.H.: Contemporary Hopi food intake patterns. Ecol. Food Nutr. *6:* 159–173 (1977).
LaChance, P.: A commentary on the new FDA nutrition labeling regulations. Nutr. Today *January/February:* 18–22 (1973).
Lappe, F.: Diet for a small planet; 10th anniversary ed. (Ballantine Books, New York 1982).
Lappe, F.; Collins, J.: Food first: beyond the myth of scarcity (Houghton-Mifflin, Boston 1977).
Leiss, W.: The limits to satisfaction: an essay on the problem of needs and commodities (University of Toronto Press, Toronto 1976).
Leslie, J.: Mass media for nutrition education (US Aid, Washington 1977).

Levy, S.R.; Everson, B.K.; Walberg, H.J.: Nutrition education research: an interdisciplinary evaluation and review. Hlth Educ. Q. *7:* 107–126 (1980).

Lewin, K.: Field theory in social science (Harper, New York 1951).

Lewis, M.W.: Women and food: an annotated bibliography on family food production, preservation and improved nutrition (Office of Women in Development, US Agency for International Development, Washington).

Longacre, D.J.: Nutrition and development. Development Monogr. Ser. 4 (Menonite Central Committee, Akron 1978).

Mahoney, M.J.; Thoresen, C.E.: Self-control: power to the person (Brooks/Cole, Monterey 1974).

Maslow, A.H.: Towards a psychology of being (Van Nostrand, Princeton 1968).

Mayer, J.: Can you tell the contents by the label? Family Hlth *January:* 18–19 (1971).

McBride, S.: Many voices, one world: towards a new more just and efficient world. International Commission for the Study of Communication Problems (Kogan Page, London 1980).

McGuire, W.J.: Conceptualizing attitudes and attitude change for nutritional research and education; in Sims, MacNeil, Attitude theory and measurement in food and nutrition research. Proc. Symp., Pennsylvania State University, University Park 1980, pp. 1–19.

McKenzie, J.C.; Mumford, P.: The evaluation of nutrition education programmes: a review of the present situation. Wld Rev. Nutr. Diet., vol. 5, pp. 21–31 (Karger, Basel 1965).

McNaughton, J.W.: A review of the activities of the FAO in nutrition education and training 1949–1977; in Sinclair, Howat, World nutrition and nutrition education, pp. 156–166 (Oxford University Press, Oxford/UNESCO, Paris 1980).

Mead, M.: Cultural patterning of nutritionally relevant behavior. J. Am. diet. Ass. *25:* 677–680 (1949).

Meyer, A.J.; Nash, J.D.; McAlister, A.; Maccoby, N.; Farguhar, J.W.: Skills training in a cardiovascular health education campaign. J. consult. clin. Psychol. *48:* 129–142 (1980).

Molitor, G.T.T.: The food system in the 1980s. J. Nutr. Educ. *12:* suppl. 1, pp. 103–111 (1980).

Moore, J.L.: Nutrition education: propagandizing vs. merchandizing. Speech at the Society for Nutrition Education Annual Meet., Minneapolis 1978.

Morse, W.; Sims, L.S.; Guthrie, H.A.: Mothers' compliance with physicians' recommendations on infant feeding. J. Am. diet. Ass. *75:* 140–148 (1979).

Mosio, M.: Personal communication (1982).

Nestor, J.; Griffiths, M.; Sharp, L.: Catalogue of mass media and support materials for nutrition in developing countries (International Nutrition Communication Service Education Development Center, Newton, in press).

Nestor, J.P.; Glotzer, J.A. (eds.): Teaching nutrition. A review of programs and research (Abt Books, Cambridge 1981).

Nutrition and Your Health: Dietary guidelines for Americans. Home and Garden Bull. No. 232 (US Department of Agriculture and US Department of Health and Human Services, 1980).

NERP: Nutrition Education Resources Project (Teachers College, Columbia University, New York 1982).

Office of Science and Technology Policy, Joint Subcommittee on Human Nutrition Research: Federally supported human nutrition research, training and education: Update for the 1980s. III. Nutrition education research and professional personnal needs for nutrition education of professionals and the public (Office of Science and Technology, Washington 1981).

Oliver, R.L.; Berger, P.K.: A path analysis of preventive health care decision models. J. Consumer Res. *6:* 113–122 (1979).

Olson, C.M.; Gillespie, A.H. (eds.): Proceedings of the workshop on nutrition education research: applying principles from the behavioral sciences. J. Nutr. Educ. *13:* suppl. 1 (1981).

Pelto, G.H.: Anthropological contributions to nutrition education research. J. Nutr. Educ. *13:* suppl., pp. 2–8 (1981a).

Pelto, G.H.: Perspectives on infant feeding: decision-making and ecology. Food Nutr. Bull. *3:* 17–29 (1981b).

Potter, J.M.: People of plenty, economic abundance and the American character (University of Chicago Press, Chicago 1958).

Rasmuson, M.: Current practice and future directions of nutrition education in developing countries: a research and policy assessment. AED Paper prepared for the Office of Nutrition and the Office of Education and Human Resources, Technical Assistance Bureau, AID, Washington 1977.

Rethinking food and nutrition education under changing socio-economic conditions. Food Nutr. Bull. *2:* 23–28 (1980).

Richmond, F.W.: The role of the federal government in nutrition education. J. Nutr. Educ. *9:* 150–151 (1977).

Rifkind, S.: Personal communication (1982).

Ringen, K.: Norway's nutrition and food policy overview, results and future directions; in McLaren, Nutrition in the community (Wiley, New York, 1983).

Ritenbaugh, C.: An anthropological perspective on nutrition. J. Nutr. Educ. *13:* suppl., pp. 12–15 (1981).

Roberts, H.: Intensive food production on a human scale (Ecology Action of the Mid-Peninsula, Palo Alto 1982).

Roddy, N.: Things go better with coconuts – program strategies in Micronesia. J. Nutr. Educ. *10:* 19–22 (1978).

Rogers, B.: The domestication of woman: discrimination in developing societies (Tanistock, London 1980).

Rogers, C.R.: Freedon to learn (Merrill, Columbus 1969).

Ross, M.L.: What's happening to food labeling? J. Am. diet. Ass. *64:* 262–267 (1974).

Rozin, P.: The selection of foods by rats, humans and other animals; in Rosenblatt, Hinde, Beer, Shaw, Advances in the study of behavior (Academic Press, New York 1976).

Sampson, N. (ed.): Farmland or wasteland: a time to choose (Rodale Press, Emmaus 1981).

Santos, W.; Lopes, N.; Barbosa, J.J.; Chaves, D.; Valente, J.C. (eds.): Nutrition and food science present knowledge and utilization, vol. 2 (Plenum Press, New York 1981).

Schachter, S.: Some extraordinary facts about obese humans and rats. Am. Psychol. *26:* 129–144 (1971).

Schuftan, C.: Ethics, ideology and nutrition. Food Policy *7:* 159–164 (1982).
Shack, K.W. (ed.): Teaching nutrition in developing countries or, the joys of eating dark green leaves (Meals for Millions Foundation, Santa Monica 1977).
Shelley, C.: Nutrition education in the Northern territory. Commonwealth Department of Health, Report of the National Nutrition Education Conf., pp. 40–54 (Commonwealth Department of Health, Canberra 1981).
Sims, L.S.: Dietary status of lactating women. II. Relation of nutritional knowledge and attitudes to nutrient intake. J. Am. diet. Ass. *73:* 147–154 (1978).
Sims, L.S.: Overview: nutrition education research in the policy arena; in Sims, Light, Directions for nutrition education research – the Penn State Conf. Proc., pp. 9–24 (Pennsylvania State University, University Park 1980a).
Sims, L.S.: Measuring nutrition-related attitudes: state of the art; in Sims, MacNeil, Attitude theory and measurement in food and nutrition research. Proc. Symp., pp. 69–76 (Pennsylvania State University, University Park 1980b).
Sims, L.S.; Light, L.: Directions for nutrition education research – the Penn State Conf. Proc. (USA and Pennsylvania State University, University Park 1980).
Sims, L.S.; MacNeil, J.H. (eds.): Attitude theory and measurement in food and nutrition research. Proc. Symp. (Agricultural Conf. Coordinator, Pennsylvania State University, University Park 1980).
Sinclair, H.M.; Howat, G.R.: World nutrition and nutrition education (Oxford University Press, Oxford/UNESCO, Paris 1980).
Skinner, B.F.: Science and human behavior (Macmillan, New York 1953).
Skinner, B.F.: Beyond freedom and dignity (Knopf, New York 1971).
Smith, K.W.; Nelson, S.K.; O'Hara, J.J.: Food for thought project, final report. Office of Policy, Planning and Evaluation, Food and Nutrition Service, US Department of Agriculture (Am. Institutes of Research, Cambridge 1982).
Society for Nutrition Education: Inside front cover: current volume. J. Nutr. Educ. *15* (1983).
Spitze, H.T.: Curriculum materials and learning at the high school level. J. Nutr. Educ. *8:* 59–61 (1976).
Srinivasan, L.: Perspectives on nonformal adult learning (World Education, New York 1977).
St. Pierre, R.G.: Specifying outcomes in nutrition education evaluation. J. Nutr. Educ. *14:* 49–51 (1982).
St. Pierre, R.G.; Resmovic, V.: An overview of the national nutrition education and training program evaluation. J. Nutr. Educ. *14:* 61–66 (1982).
Staff of the Select Committee on Nutrition and Human Needs, United States Senate: Dietary Goals for the United States (US Government Printing Office, Washington 1977).
State of the Environment, A report from the Conservation Foundation (Conservation Foundation, Washington 1982).
Stunkard, A.J.; Penick, S.J.: Behavior modification in the treatment of obesity. Archs gen. Psychiat. *36:* 801–806 (1979).
Sullivan, A.D.; Schwartz, N.E.: Attitudes, knowledge, and practices related to diet and cardiovascular disease. J. Can. diet. Ass. *42:* 169–177 (1981).
Swope, M.R.: A review of nutrition education research. Nutrition Education Research Project, 30 p. mimeo (Teachers College, Columbia University, New York 1982).

Szczygiel, M.: Influence of socio-economic and other factors on nutritional habits in Poland. Biblthca Nutr. Dieta, No. 20, pp. 92–104 (Karger, Basel 1974).

Talmadge, H.; Hughes, M.; Eash, M.J.: The role of evaluation research in nutrition educating. J. Nutr. Educ. *10:* 169–172 (1978).

Tepley, L.J.: Conference on nutrition education. Am. J. clin. Nutr. *26:* 678–681 (19739.

Terreri, N.J.: An integrated development approach to solving rural nutrition problems, or soft is beatiful; in Shack, Teaching nutrition in developing countries or, the joys of eating dark green leaves (Meals for Millions Foundation, Santa Monica 1977).

Tinker, I.: New technologies for food-related activities: an equity strategy; in Dauber, Cain, Women and technological change in developing countries (Westview Press, Boulder 1980).

Truswell, A.S.: Changing concepts of healthy diets in prosperous communities; in Sinclair, Howat, World nutrition and nutrition education, pp. 44–50 (Oxford University Press, Oxford/UNESCO, Paris 1980).

Tudge, C.: The famine business (Penguin Books, New York 1977).

Tudge, C.: Future food: politics, philosophy and recipes for the 21st century (Harmony Books, New York 1980).

Tyebjee, T.T.: Affirmative disclosure of nutrition information and consumers' food preferences: a review. J. Consumer Affairs *13:* 206–223 (1979).

Tyler, R.W.: Basic principles of curriculum and instruction (University of Chicago Press, Chicago 1950).

Ullrich, H.D.: Towards a national educaiton policy. J. Nutr. Educ. *11:* 60 (1979).

UNESCO: Statistical Yearbook (UNESCO, Paris 1981).

UNESCO: Nutrition education: curriculum planning and selectee case studies. Science and Technology Document Ser. 3, ED.82/WS/78 (UNESCO, Paris 1982).

UNICEF hits Nestlé on code interpretation. CNI Weekly Report *XII:* 7 (1982).

United Nations Development Programs: Rural women's participation in development. Evaluation Study No. 3 (UNDP, New York 1980).

United States Department of State: The global 2000 report to the president, vol. 1 (US Government Printing Office, Washington 1980).

Ward, W.B.: Determining health education impact through proxy measures of behavior change. Health Education, *May/June:* 19–23 (1981).

Watson, J.B.: Psychology as the behaviorist views it. Psychol. Rev. *20:* 158–177 (1913).

Webb, R.E.; Ballweg, A.; Pougere, W.: Combining nutrition education with agricultural training in Haiti. J. Nutr. Educ. *14:* 133–184 (1982).

Whitehead, F.E.: Nutrition education research. Wld Rev. Nutr. Diet., vol. 17, pp. 91–149 (Karger, Basel 1973).

Wolf, R.: The role of evaluation in nutrition education; in Sinclair, Howat, World nutrition and nutrition education, pp. 109–113 (Oxford University Press, Oxford/UNESCO, Paris 1980).

Worlsey, A.: Thought for food: investigations of cognitive aspects of food. Econology Food Nutr. *9:* 65–80 (1980).

Yarbrough, P.: Communication theory and nutrition education research. J. Nutr. Educ. *13:* suppl., 16–27 (1981).

Yudkin, J.: Introduction; in Yudkin, Diet of man: needs and wants (Applied Science publishers, London 1978).

Yudkin, J.: Objectives and methods in nutrition education – Let's start again. J. hum. Nutr., Lond. *35:* 205–213 (1981).

Zeitlin, M.: Directions for the evaluation of nutrition education; in Shack, Teaching nutrition in developing countries or the joys of eating dark green leaves, pp. 169–193 (Meals for Millions, Santa Monica 1977).

Zeitlin, M.; Formacion, C.S.: Nutrition intervention in developing countries. Study II. Nutrition education, p. 6, 18, 22, 25, 33 (Oelgeschlager, Gunn & Hain, Cambridge 1981).

J.D. Gussow, MD, Department of Nutrition Education, Teachers College, Columbia University, New York, NY 10027 (USA)

Wld Rev. Nutr. Diet., vol. 44, pp. 57–84 (Karger, Basel 1984)

Evolution of the French Diet: Nutritional Aspects

Henri Dupin, Serge Hercberg, Véronique Lagrange

Institut Scientifique et Technique de l'Alimentation du
Conservatoire National des Arts et Métiers, Paris, France

Contents

Introduction

In many countries, nutrition has changed more profoundly during the last decades than during the preceding centuries. Certain aspects of this evolution have shown themselves to be positive while other aspects are negative as they have contributed to the development of illnesses due to overweight. The rapid evolution of diet in a country and the profound change (a real upheaval) of the place of various food groups in the daily diet is of interest to all those involved in nutrition and public health.

The goal of this article is to describe the evolution of nutrition in one country, France, and to compare it with what has taken place in other industrialized nations. We shall also give figures on the consumption of different nutrients as well as the differences that can be noted according to regions and those that exist between socio-economic categories.

The upheavals noted in the dietary habits of wealthy countries during the last 50 years are due to multiple causes: the change in the production methods in agriculture and breeding, the development of preserving techniques and commercial techniques, and the rise in purchasing power. All these have contributed to increasing the availability of food, whereas the improvement in living conditions has led to a lessening of energy needs while encouraging the individual to consume more.

We have at our disposal several sources of information to study and analyze the evolution of the diet of the French population:

The Ministry of Agriculture has published for over 60 years summaries of the quantities of nutrients placed on the market for human consumption. The Central Service for Investigation and Statistical Studies gives detailed information taking into account imports, exports, and uses other than dietary. These figures, although they deal with availabiliy per capita rather than actual human consumption, are very interesting as they allow us to follow an evolution over a long period [16a, b].

The FAO (Food and Agriculture Organization) and the OECD (Organization for Economic Cooperation and Development) publish important documents [9, 18]. For the quantities concerning France, they use, to a large extent, the figures issued by the Ministry of Agriculture. We have used the FAO and OECD publications to prepare the tables and charts which compare for a given nutrient our country with other industrialized countries.

The INSEE (National Institute for Statistics and Economic Studies) has carried out since 1965 an 'investigation on the diet of the French'. 10,000 households are surveyed and this sample, representative of the French population, is renewed in totality each year. The results are analyzed to give figures on average per capita consumption for all of France, but they are also analyzed according to region, to level of urbanization, as well as to the socio-economic category of the head of the household [15, 26, 27, 32]. However, this survey is limited to household consumption within the home and does not take into account either meals taken out of the home or permanent organizations such as the army, etc. Other surveys, although less broad, allow us to fill this gap.

The professional organizations of the food and agricultural sector of the economy have precise statistics on the production and consumption of one nutrient or group of nutrients (grains, dairy products, oils and margarines, sugar, etc.). Another source of information are the dietary surveys carried out by nutritionists and epidemiologists. They are often of great interest for the knowledge of dietary consumption (as opposed to dietary purchases or availabilities) but they usually deal with fairly small samples of the population. Studies on dietary motivation and behaviour allow us to better grasp the attitude of the consumer to a product or to a technological innovation. The National Institute for Agricultural Research has research groups studying the economics and sociology of diet [3, 14].

The various sources of information do not always give us identical figures for a given nutrient and period. We can sometimes note differences which are due, to a large part, to the fact that the chosen definitions or criteria are not exactly identical. However, in using all available data, we observe that the series of figures which allow us to follow over the years the evolution of consumption are very comparable. And in this article, it is precisely these evolutionary tendencies in one country – France – that we wish to present.

These following subjects are dealt with below: (1) The consumption of nutrients which have as a principal characteristic their carbohydrate input: on the one hand grains, starches, pulses, and on the other hand, fruits, and finally beetroot or cane sugar (saccharose). (2) The consumption of meat, fish, eggs, and cheese and the study of the respective place in the daily diet of proteins of vegetable origin and those of animal origin. (3) The place occupied by lipids in meals and the nature of these lipids. (4) Alcoholic beverages.

Evolution of the Consumption of Foods Whose Principal Characteristic Is the Input of Carbohydrates

Nutrients Rich in Starch and Other Complex Carbohydrates

Bread. The average daily per capita consumption of bread in France is shown in table I. One can note that in one century bread consumption has decreased by more than two thirds and that in 40 years it has decreased by more than half [7]. Of course, these figures are only averages and hide

Table I. Evolution of bread consumption in France (g/person/day)

1880	about 600	1967	224
1910	about 500	1972	187
1936	325	1980	172

Table II. Evolution of potato consumption in France (kg/person/year)

1925	178	1975	91
1955	125	1980	84.5
1965	105		

important differences between rural and urban populations as well as the various socio-economic categories [23, 25].

The consumption of packaged toasted bread increased greatly from 1950 to 1974. Since then it has seemed to stabilize while the consumption of packaged grilled or braised bread, packaged sandwich bread and pastries, is still increasing. But this is far from compensating the decrease in the use of bread. The total quantitiy of wheat (hard and soft wheat) used for human consumption has gone from 99 kg per person per year in 1960 to 74 kg in 1978.

Potatoes. The consumption of potatoes decreased by half in France between 1925 and 1980 (table II). There are here again large differences according to regions [25, 26] and according to socio-economic categories [26], as we shall see further on. A greater and greater proportion of potato purchases is taking the form of industrially modified products (peeled potatoes, fried potatoes) or in processed products (flake potatoes for quick mashed potatoes, croquettes and potato cakes, prepared dishes). This will most likely lead during the coming years to the slowing or stopping of the decrease in consumption.

Pulses. Their consumption has considerably diminished in France (table III). However, two factors have slowed this fall: pulses are used in making processed foods. Others (beans and chick peas) are found in North African recipes whose use is spreading in France and red beans which are being used in exotic preparations such as Mexican salad.

Some vegetables have almost disappeared from the diet of French families either because of their lack of taste or appreciation or because they

Table III. Evolution of pulse consumption in France (kg/person/year)

1925	7.3	1978	1.7
1970	2.3	1980	1.4

Table IV. Evolution of sugar consumption in France (kg/person/year)

1850	3	1953	26
1910	17	1973	36
1920	19	1980	36
1935–1940	22		

needed long preparation. The same may be said for some foods rich in starch. In several regions of the centre and southwest of the country as well as in Haute Provence and Corsica, chestnuts used to be a staple food and were eaten almost daily during several months of the year [7]. It is estimated that the harvest a century ago was 500,000 t whereas presently it is 15,000 t. The festivities which marked the beginning of the chestnut harvest are still celebrated in several towns in Provence, but the present generation has no idea of the importance that this farinaceous food had in the family diet.

On the whole, consumption in France of these different foods rich in complex carbohydrates (in particular starch) containing protein of vegetable origin and fibre has fallen considerably during the last decades [7, 19]. This phenomenon is not specifically French, as identical situations can be seen in most of the industrialized countries (fig. 1).

Today grains account for only 20–25% of the daily energy input in industrialized countries and roots and tubercules for only 5–6% (on the other hand, as we all know, in many developing countries grains and/or roots and tubercules account alone for 70–85% of the energy input).

Foods Supplying Rapid Absorption Carbohydrates

Evolution of Sugar Consumption. In France, we are speaking primarily of saccharose. Aside from the small quantities contained in fruits and vegetables, this saccharose comes on the one hand from the cultivation in France of beets and on the other hand from the cultivation of sugar cane in overseas departments (Martinique and Guadeloupe in the West Indies and the Island of Réunion in the Indian Ocean). The average consumption of sugar in France is shown in table IV. It has considerably increased since the

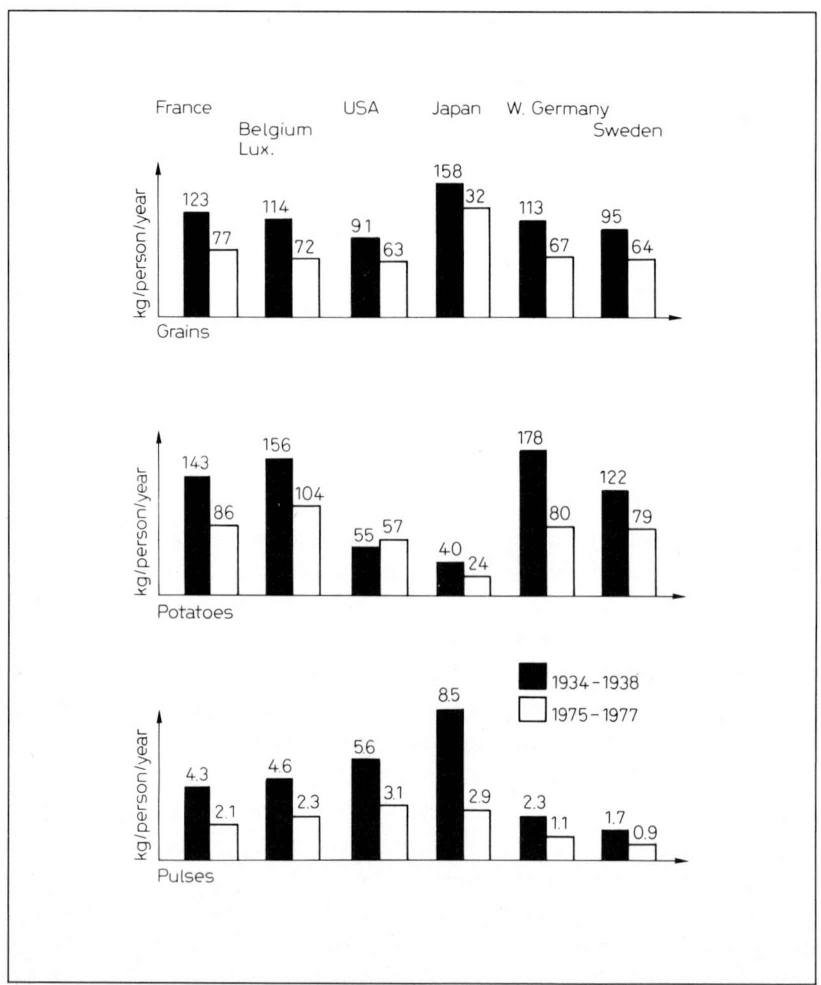

Fig. 1. Evolution of the grain, potato and pulses consumption (kg/person/year) in some industrialized countries. Two periods have been compared: 1934–1938 and 1975–1977 according to FAO data [9].

beginning of the century but seems to have stabilized over the last decade around 36 kg/person/year. It is important to distinguish between the consumption of raw sugar which has decreased over several years, and the amounts included in industrial foods and drinks which has considerably increased.

Table V. Some industrial uses of sugar in France

	Thousands of tons		
	1960	1970	1979
Chocolates and sweets	137	188	217
Biscuits, packaged toasted bread, diet foods, desserts	86	125	117
Soft drinks	41	98	138
Sirups	18	58	110
Jam and canned fruits	51	78	89
Pastry	21	24	57
Pre-sweetened yogurts, puddings, and dessert creams	3	19	37
Ice creams	6	13	30
Canned vegetables	2	3	5

Globally, including the adding of sugar to wine, the use of sugar by industries has gone from 449,500 t in 1960 to 962,000 t in 1979, thereby more than doubling in 20 years with very great increases these last years in certain areas (table V). This 'indirect' sugar input is hardly perceived or even completely ignored by consumers. It is particularly high among children and adolescents, great users of sweetened drinks, pastries and dessert puddings, although this does not appear in the figures for average national consumption.

There has been a similar evolution of sugar consumption in many industrialized countries over the last decades (fig. 2). For some of these countries per capita sugar consumption is greater than ours. This is the case in Sweden, Canada and the USA, in Great Britain, in Switzerland, in Australia, etc. In the USA, along with saccharose consumption, annual per capita consumption of glucose from corn is 17 kg (we do not have this problem in France). The total annual per capita consumption of sugar in the USA in 1977 was 56 kg, which represented 24% of the daily energy intake. The USA, like the Scandinavian countries, have included among their nutritional goals a decrease in this consumption.

At present, the consumption of sugar-saccharose in France represents 15% of the total energy input. This level corresponds to the recommendations of a commission in the USA. But if the progression of sugar quantities used by the food industries continues at the same pace of preceding years, it is probable that this percentage will be exceeded. Certain industrial uses of sugar in France are still far from those noted in the USA (table VI).

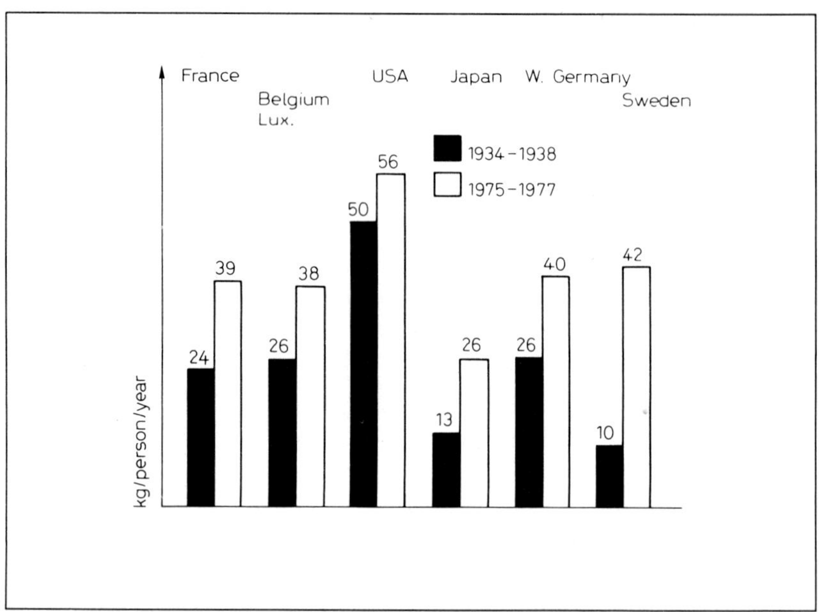

Fig. 2. Evolution of sugar consumption in various industrialized countries between 1934–1938 and 1975–1977 according to FAO data [9].

Table VI. Comparison of ice cream and soft drink consumption (1977) in France and the USA

	France litres	USA litres
Ice cream	4	23.7
Soft drinks	23	136

On the whole, the use of starches (bread and other grain products, potatoes and other farinaceous vegetables, and pulses) has greatly diminished in France, as in the other industrialized countries, while the consumption of saccharose has greatly increased. It seems to have stabilized in our country over the last decade, but the large quanties of sugar used in various prepared foods and beverages indicate that this stabilization is precarious.

Fruit as a Particular Situation. The consumption of fruit in France has greatly increased over the last decade. According to data supplied by the Ministry of Agriculture, by the INSEE, and by professional organizations, consumption has increased from 31 kg annual per capita consumption in 1951 to 52 kg in 1961, and to 72 kg in 1980.

Like all the wealthy countries, we import for our pleasure fruit from all parts of the world. This growth has been promoted by modern techniques of preservation and by the development of air freight. The poorest nations, even while suffering from famine, continue to export fruit to the wealthy countries. During the drought of 1971–1973 and the great famine which followed, African countries (Sahel region) continued to produce strawberries to export to Europe. Comparable situations exist between some Central American countries and the USA. We, as wealthy populations, are able to have poor countries produce our luxury foods for our pleasure, even when these countries are lacking in the basic needs. However, to concentrate on this problem is not the goal of this article.

It must be noted that the consumption of fruit preserves and canned fruit is, in France, much lower than that in Canada or in the USA, as the French do not like these processed fruits. In recent years, frozen fruit has had a modest acceptance but, in general, in our country when we speak of fruit we mean fresh fruit.

Evolution of the Consumption of Meat, Fish, Eggs, and Dairy Foods – Change in the Use of Proteins of Animal Origin and Proteins of Vegetable Origin

Meat

The low consumption of meat in the French countryside in the 17th, 18th and beginning of the 19th centuries has been mentioned in several works. *Vauban,* France's greatest military engineer, described in his work, *Dîme Royale,* the state of the kingdom of France. This work, published in 1707 and containing much information on life in the provinces, was seized and condemned on the king's order. As an example one can read in regard to the region of Vezelay: '... the populace does not eat meat three times in 1 year ...' In 1791, *Lavoisier,* in his work *De la Richesse Territoriale du Royaume de France,* maintained that a large number of the inhabitants of the countryside did not eat meat, except during the celebration of Easter and marriage ceremonies. We could cite many other works and many other

Table VII. Evolution of the average quantity of meat intended for human consumption (all meats including poultry) (kg/person/year)

1840	20	1959	69
1900	30	1964	76
1922	41	1969	84
1938	47	1974	90
1952	60	1980	110

Table VIII. Evolution of the amount of meat used (kg/person/year). These figures are based on the weight of carcasses as delivered to butcher shops and to companies serving food – the amounts actually consumed are less

	Pork	Beef	Poultry	Veal	Mutton	Horse meat
1960	21.4	18.5	9.1	7.5	2.5	2.3
1980	37.2	26.2	16.7	6.9	4.1	1.7

observers, but this would become tiresome. Analyzing as precisely as possible that evolution of meat consumption according to the available data, the figures shown in table VII give us an idea of the changes over a period of 140 years.

These figures, supplied by the Central Service for Research and Statistical Studies of the Ministry of Agriculture [16a, b], correspond to the weight of carcasses (minus the fat removed during butchering) and takes into account exports and imports as well as the changes in the French population during the years considered. These figures are greater than the actual annual per capita meat consumption as the butcher, followed by the housewife or the food service personnel, eliminates certain parts, and finally the consumer leaves on his plate the fattiest or thoughest part. But what is most interesting is the evolution of consumption, and in this area everything shows that the average meat consumption has doubled during the last 50 years [3, 7, 16a, b].

The increase in meat consumption in France includes all meats, with the exception of veal (high-priced) and horse meat (table VIII). Veal consumption has slightly diminished between 1960 and 1980, but the French

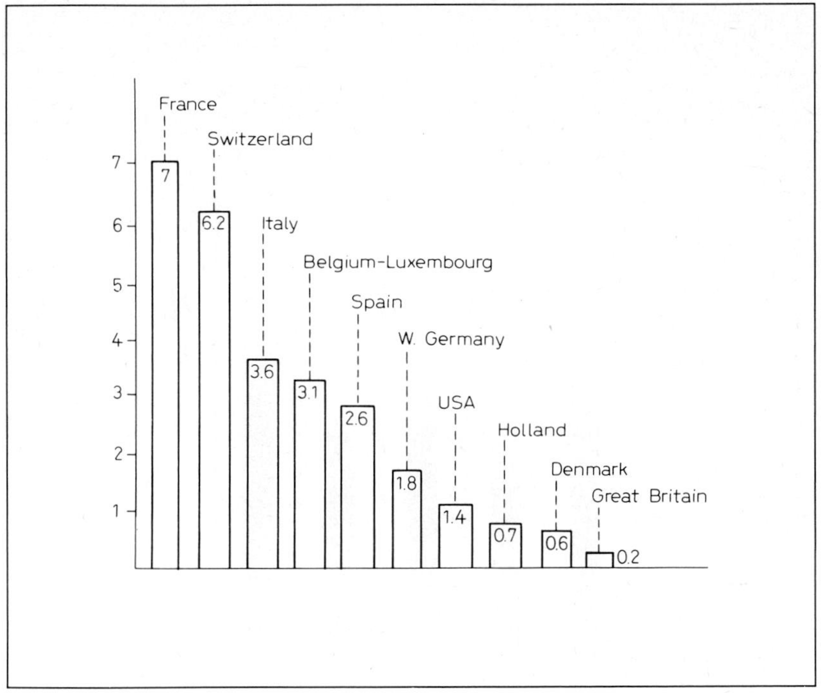

Fig. 3. Veal (kg/person/year) consumption in 1978 according to OECD data [18].

are still large consumers of it. This behaviour is not very logical as it is not economically very profitable to slaughter animals which are far from having reached their maximum development. Figure 3 shows the difference in consumption between countries, but we must note that comparisons are made difficult by the fact that the definition of veal (in comparison to baby beef) is not identical from one country to another.

The amount of poultry consumed per person per year in France has almost doubled during the last 20 years. The industrial production of chicken dates from more than 20 years ago. The production of turkeys is more recent and quail production seems to be headed for a rapid development.

Concerning beef, 60% of purchases are made up of roasting or grilling cuts coming from the hind quarters of the animal. The French appreciate less those cuts requiring slow cooking (which come mostly from the fore-

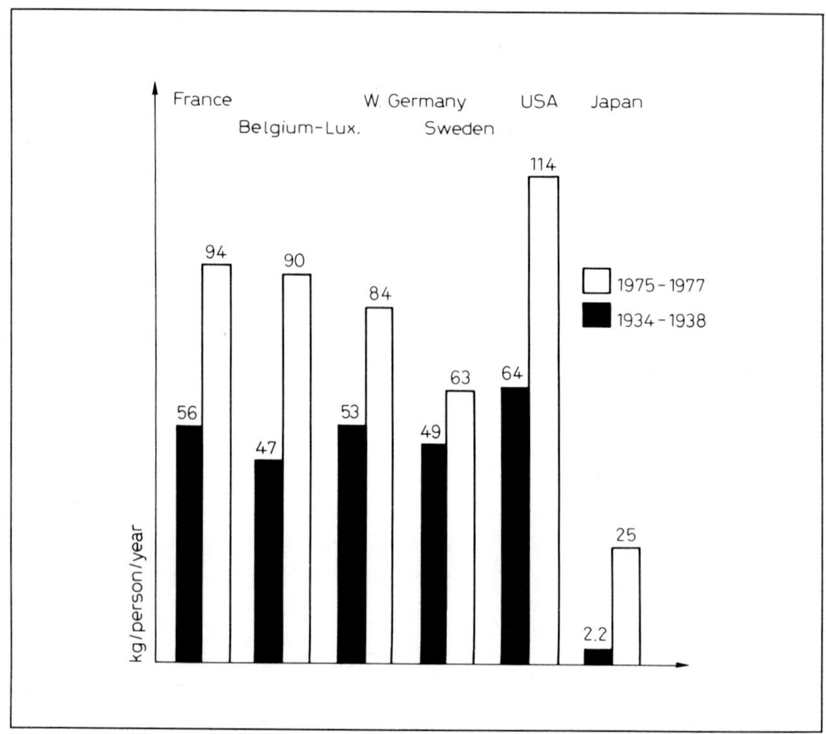

Fig. 4. Evolution of meat consumption (kg/person/year) in some industrialized countries between 1934–1938 and 1975–1977 according to FAO data [9].

quarters of the animal). Industrial products which use these cuts of lesser gastronomical quality have an increasing market thanks mainly to frozen preparations, but in this area, France is behind countries like Germany and the USA.

The increase in meat consumption observed in France during these last decades can be seen in all the industrialized countries and most particularly in Japan which consumed meat in very small quantities 40 years ago (fig. 4). Although global consumption (all meat considered) has risen in all these countries, there remain large variations in the different types of meat consumed (table IX). Meat consumption is much greater in industrialized countries than in developing countries (from 3 to 50 times greater according to the country considered).

Table IX. Consumption of different types of meat in some industrialized countries in 1978 [18] (kg/person/year)

	Beef	Veal	Pork	Poultry	Horse meat
France	25	7	37.2	15.9	1.8
USA	54.9	1.4	28.1	26	–
Denmark	16.3	0.6	45.6	8.4	0.4
W. Germany	22.3	1.8	55.7	9.9	0.1
Italy	20.3	3.6	21.3	17.3	1.2
Spain	10.3	2.6	22.9	20.9	0.2

Table X. Evolution of proteins of animal origin in the total protein input of the daily diet in France

	%		%
1880	27	1955	51
1920	39	1975	64
1935	45	1980	71

Other Sources of Protein of Animal Origin

Over the last years, the increase in the consumption of fish in France has stayed very slight and has diminished for fresh, salted, dried, or smoked fish. The increase in consumption has been in canned or frozen fish.

The consumption of eggs (including the use in food industries) has gone from 10.5 kg/person/year in 1959 to 13.1 kg in 1978. This consumption is less than that of the USA (16.5 kg/person/year) or that of West Germany (17.1 kg/person/year). Measures in the USA aimed at improving public health have suggested a reduction in egg consumption and a certain decrease has been noted.

In France, the use of milk as a beverage (all forms of preservation included) has diminished, particularly during the last 20 years, while the amounts used by industry have increased (yogurts, dessert puddings). Cheese consumption [16a, b] has more than doubled during the last 20 years, going from 8.8 kg/person/year in 1959 to 18.8 kg/person/year in 1980, which comes to an average of 50 g/person/day. As we all know, the French are very proud of the richness and diversity of cheeses.

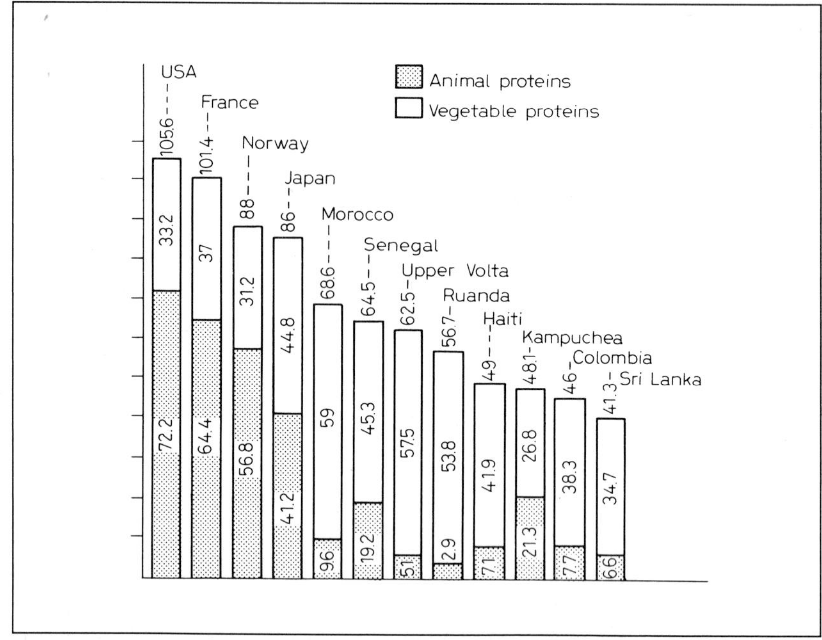

Fig. 5. Average consumption of proteins of animal and vegetable origin (g/person/day) according to FAO data [9].

The study of the respective evolution of consumption in France of various foods providing proteins shows a small increase in protein consumption over the last four decades. The French today eat a lot fewer proteins of vegetable origin (as supplied by bread and other grain products and pulses) than preceding generations. On the other hand, they eat more proteins of animal origin (as supplied by meat, eggs, and dairy products) [7, 19]. A century ago, proteins of animal origin accounted for 27% of the total daily protein intake. Today they account for 71% (table X). Obviously, this represents a considerable change.

The food consumption models of industrialized countries are characterized by a large protein input of which more than 60%, and in some cases more than 70%, is of animal origin. The level of protein input in developing countries depends to a large extent on the staple diet (grains or tubercules) but the greater part of these proteins are of vegetable origin; figure 5 shows the differences between some countries.

Evolution of the Part of Lipids in the Daily Diet and the Change in Their Nature

Place of Lipids in Total Energy Input in France

To a greater extent than with any other nutrient, we must distinguish between the 'quantities used in human nutrition' and the 'quantities actually consumed', and therefore must keep in mind certain facts [7, 11, 12]: (1) Only a part of the lipids present in foods or in dishes is actually ingested. In fact, the fats used for salad dressings and sauces both prepared in the family or industrially are not totally consumed. As for deep frying fats, they are discarded after a certain number of uses. Also, many people leave on their plates the fattiest pieces of meats or sausage products. It is estimated that the proportion of lipids thus discarded is approximately 10% as no more precise study has been made. (2) The 'food composition tables' actually used in France show quantities for meat lipids which are greater than the lipids in meat presently consumed.

Estimated with these reservations, lipid consumption has globally increased by 60% between 1934–1938 and 1975–1977 to go from 92 to 145 g/person/day. An important fact is that 71% of these consumed lipids are presently of animal origin. This increase is still continuing, but slowly. This evolution is due to the following facts: (1) Over the last decade, the French population has reduced its global energy input, this reduction being mainly in bread, grain products, potatoes, and with very little reduction in lipids [4, 19]. (2) We use less food cooked in water, fewer soups, more fried foods or foods cooked with fats, and more salads whose dressing includes lipids. (3) The increase in meat consumption is inexorably followed by a greater lipid input, depending on whether fatty parts are discarded. (4) The consumption of butter has increased, going from 7.7 kg/person/year in 1959 to 9.3 kg in 1981, which represents 20.8–25.5 g/day [12, 16a, b]. But here again, these averages hide great differences between individuals, socio-economic categories, and regions. Margarine consumption in France is clearly less than that in Germany or Holland but is slowly increasing, from 3.06 kg/person/year in 1968 to 3.80 kg in 1981.

Up to 1950–1955, the average consumption in France held to the limit suggested by nutritionists for the amount of energy supplied by lipids (not more than 30–33% of the total daily energy input). Before the First World War, between 1880 and 1913, lipids accounted for approximately 22% of energy input, and between the two wars, from 1920 to 1939, for about 28%. But at present in France, the amount of energy supplied by lipids represents

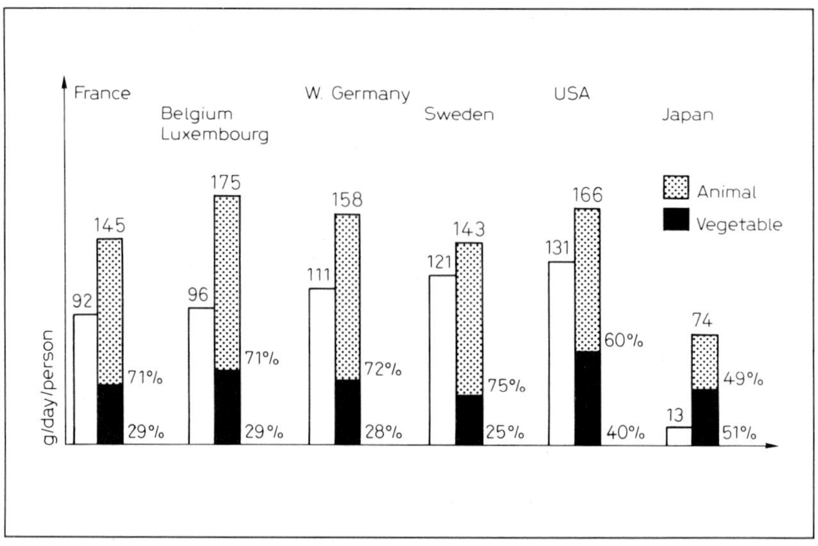

Fig. 6. Average lipid consumption (g/person/day) in some industrialized countries, comparing two periods, 1934–1938 and 1975–1977 according to FAO data [9].

42% of the total energy input of the diet [7, 8, 19]. This is mainly due to the increase in lipid intake through meats, butter, cheese and eggs. It is therefore lipids of animal origin (which have a high level of saturated fatty acids) which have increased.

In France today, naturally occurring lipids (as opposed to added fats) account for 66% of the total lipids in the diet [12]. A similar evolution has occurred in the industrialized countries although the increase in lipid consumption has obviously been less in those countries which already had a high intake 40 years ago (USA, Sweden). However, Japan, which had a very low level of consumption 40 years ago, has seen it multiplied by 6 (fig. 7).

On the whole, the evolution of the French diet from a nutritional standpoint, as in other industrialized countries, has resulted in: (1) A global decrease in energy input. Our style of life has changed and the energy necessary for manual labour and thermoregulation has been considerably reduced. We have reduced our energy input, but less than our energy use [4, 8]. (2) A large diversification of our diet, which has led to a better mix of the different food groups in our daily diet. (3) A change in the repartition of

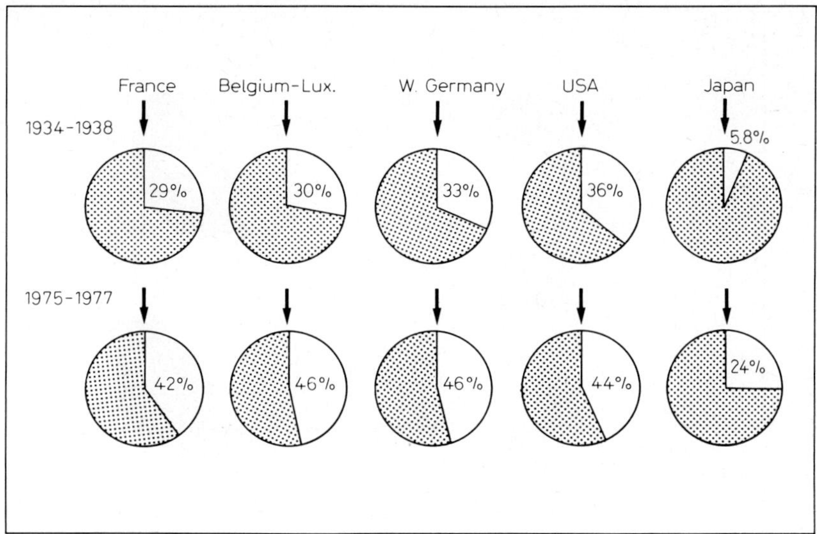

Fig. 7. Lipid share in the total energy input of the diet. Increase of lipids in total energy input in different industrialized countries, comparing the two periods 1934–1938 and 1975–1977 according to FAO data [9].

different nutrients in meeting energy needs: a decrease in carbohydrates, particularly complex carbohydrates, an increase in proteins of animal origin and a decrease in proteins of vegetable origin, an increase in lipids replacing carbohydrates, and a decrease in food fibres.

This evolution has led to a diet model quite removed from the recommendations of the majority of public health nutritionists. Persons interested in the relationship between diet and cardiovascular risk are aware that the incidence of ischaemic cardiopathies is considerably lower in France than in the USA, Canada or in the European countries of comparable living standards [5, 6, 22], while their diet is relatively similar. The reasons for this lower incidence have not yet been clearly determined.

It is interesting to try to present as fully as possible the diets of different peoples, even if the available data may be criticized. Many publications have established these comparisons between countries in the form of tables. Two of the authors have prepared a series of figures [to be published] and we are presenting one here as an example (fig. 8). It allows us to see simultaneously for each country the average energy content of the diet and the role of each of the three major energy sources in that diet [8].

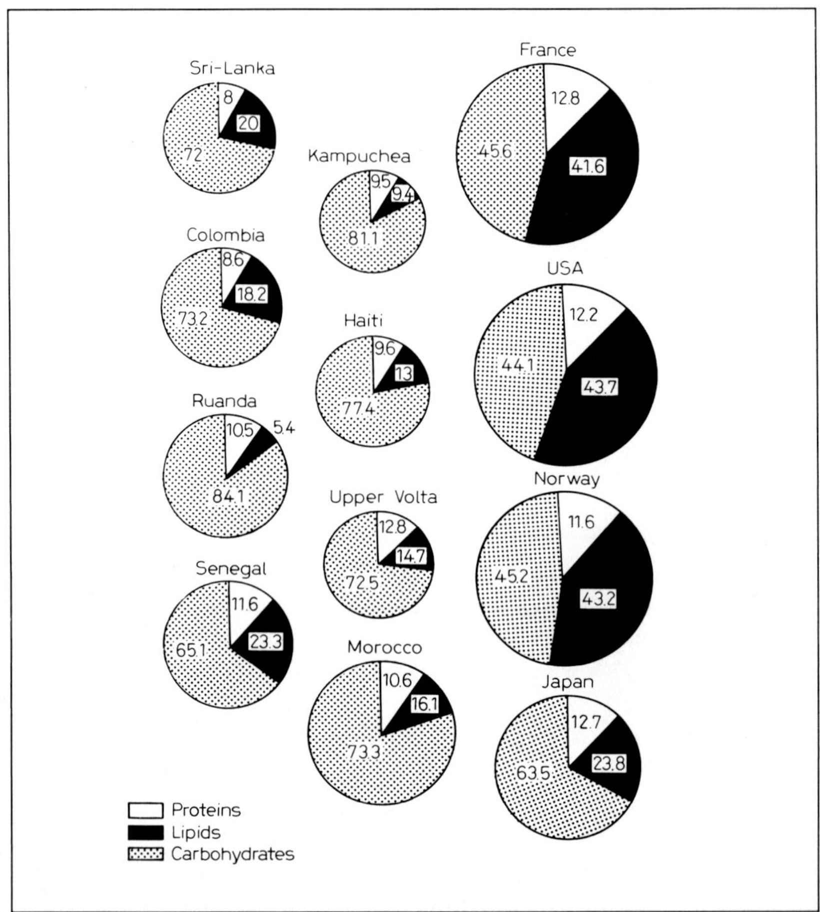

Fig. 8. Respective part in the diet of carbohydrates, lipids and proteins. The diameter of the circle is proportional to the average energy input in the diet of the country. The energy input from alcoholic beverages is expressed in carbohydrates according to FAO data [9].

Problems Caused by Beverages

The average consumption of wine in France has decreased from 172 l/person of over 20 years of age in 1940 to 127 litres in 1960 and to 98 litres in 1978. However, the study of the 'average' is of limited value due to the considerable differences between individual consumption. In com-

Table XI. Evolution of consumption in France of various distilled beverages (hectolitres)

	Anis beverages	Whisky, gin, vodka	Liqueurs
1970	385,000	66,700	60,000
1975	528,000	107,000	97,000

Table XII. Evolution of pure alcohol consumption between 1950–1952 and 1975–1976 (litres/person over 20 years of age/year)

	Pure alcohol consumption		
	1950/1952	1975/1976	difference, %
Wine			
France	17.6	16.5	− 6.2
Portugal	12.9	14.1	+ 9.3
Italy	9.4	12.7	+ 35
Beer			
W. Germany	3.6	12.5	+ 247
Czechoslovakia	4.9	9.2	+ 87
Denmark	4	9.2	+ 130
Spirits			
E. Germany	1.9	8.3	+ 330
Yugoslavia	2.7	8.9	+ 230
Holland	1.9	8.3	+ 337

parison, beer consumption was 50.6 l/person of over 20 years of age in 1956, 59.5 litres in 1966 and 71.3 litres in 1976. The quantities of alcoholic beverages and hard liquors has also increased (table XI).

In spite of the slight decrease in consumption noted these last years, France is still the country with the highest consumption of alcohol per person. This has a very strong influence on morbidity and on mortality. In our country, alcohol is responsible for at least 40,000 deaths per year. In addition, for those people who drink moderately and will never be alcoholics, alcoholic beverages have the drawback of adding to an already too high energy input.

In various countries, epidemiological studies have sought to identify alcohol as a risk factor in cancer of the upper digestive passages, and in particular the oesophagus. In France, a study carried out in Brittany [31] has given very definite conclusions on this question and on the particularly high risk of the alcohol-tobacco combination.

Those countries which are traditionally 'wine consumers' are in general those with the highest pure alcohol consumption per inhabitant. But during the last 25–30 years, there has been a considerable increase in alcohol consumption in those countries which traditionally drank beer or spirits (table XII).

The question arises as to whether world consumption of pure alcohol is equalizing. It should be noted that the consumption of alcohol has greatly increased in developing countries and the World Health Organization has called attention to this worrying fact.

Socio-Economic Aspects of Diet Evolution

Literature is often a good source of information on diet of the different social classes of the 19th century. Of all the authors we could cite, the best known in this area are probably *Charles Dickens* (1812–1870) for his works on the poor classes in Great Britain and, for France, *Emile Zola* (1840–1902). In *Zola's* novels, there are many passages on the proletariat's diet problems, malnutrition and scarcity of meat. *Victor Hugo,* in *Les Misérables* (published in 1862), tells the story of *Jean Valjean* who, driven by hunger, stole a loaf of bread. Society was hard on the least advantaged because the outcome of stealing of a loaf of bread was a prison sentence. All these descriptions seem to us to come from a very distant time and, in fact, the diet situation in industrial countries has fundamentally changed since the middle of the 19th century. In the 19th century the French middle class turned meals, and the daily meal, into a visible manifestation of its social position, both economic and political, and in the face of an aristocracy which had somewhat lost its influence. *Aron* [1] adds much to this subject. An abundance of dishes and the quality of service became tangible signs of social success. Other authors [29] have supplied figures on the evolution of consumption.

But the goal of this article is to consider the evolution which has taken place during the last decades. Some recently published autobiographies of people who were 10 or 12 years of age in 1910 and who have precise memories of their childhood provide us with precious evidence. On the most obvious facts is that in the proletarian class, mean was rare, the use of food very limited, and meals were monotonous. These autobiographical accounts add much to statistical studies covering the first quarter of the 20th century. Although table VII shows the global evolution of meat consumption as a national average, we must try to define this evolution for the different social classes.

Undoubtedly, diet has been democratized; and in particular, in meat consumption. We can see this in daily speech. The preoccupation of the 19th century French labourer was 'to earn his bread' and this expression was constantly repeated in political speeches. For the labourer in the years 1920–1930, and again during the period which immediately followed the Second World War, the preoccupation was 'to defend his beefsteak'. At present, demands take the form of a search for quality and worries about additives or residues present in certain foods.

As we have already seen, consumption of meat, eggs, and cheese has greatly increased over the last decade [2, 3, 7, 24, 29]. Purchasing power has increased and the costs of production have, for certain food products, decreased considerably. Today it takes two times less work hours than in 1920 for a steel worker to buy a kilogram of pork or ham. It takes ten times less work time to buy a dozen eggs. We can also look further back into the past: expressed in a Parisian labourer's work time, the price of a kilogram of bread is 150 times less than it was two centuries ago, although many factors come into this evolution, among them an increase in grain output per hectare.

In France, as in all the industrialized countries, the share of food expenditures in total household expenditures is decreasing while the share of health, leisure, and durable goods expenditures is increasing [17, 24]. We can estimate that in 1950, food expenditures amounted to 43% of household purchases and that in 1980 this percentage is only 21%[1]. In our opinion, these percentages should be considered with care as we personally think that the purchase of appliances for home preservation (refrigerators or freezers) and for the preparation of food should be included in food purchases, which would give a more exact idea of food expenditures in re-

[1] *Ernst Engel,* a German economist and statistician, established on the basis of an analysis of Belgian family budgets, four propositions known under the name of Engel's law and dealing with variations in demand as a function of family income. One must not confuse him with *Friedrich Engels,* the great socialist theoretician, although they lived at exactly the same period.

Table XIII. Diet in relation to socio-economic categories, from the INSEE survey [15] (kg/person/year)

	Farmer	Labourer	Manager	Shopkeeper/ Professional
Bread	91.49	56.42	36.91	42.24
Potatoes	66.88	61.47	44.95	51.02
Citrus fruits	18.08	23.83	30.62	35.19
Pulse	2.50	1.47	1.53	0.70
Meat (beef)	21.48	21.50	24.61	28.57
Fresh fish	5.59	4.77	6.14	8.67
Fruits	66.30	59.51	78.21	94.99

lation to other expenditures. In addition, these global rates at national level hide large disparities. There still exist large differences in consumer models according to the socio-economic category of the head of the family. And mention should be made of 'social stratification and the diet model' [14].

As we mentioned in the opening paragraphs of this article, the INSEE has conducted regularly since 1965 a 'study on household diets' with a sample of 10,000 households, newly chosen each year. This data is analyzed from a national perspective, but also regionally, or by city, or in terms of the socio-economic category of the head of the family.

In preparing table XIII, we only considered four socio-economic groups and a small number of foods because a table containing too many figures would have been unreadable. There are without doubt considerable differences between the four socio-economic categories we considered.

Some studies conducted by the Economic and Sociological Researchers of the National Institute of Agronomic Research [3, 14], or by consumer associations, or by the food industry, or by public or private institutions [13] allow a finer and more precise analysis of the differences in consumption according to social categories. As shown by *Grignon and Grignon* [14], inexpensive foods (potatoes, pasta, margarine) are much more widely used in the working classes than in the more advantaged classes.

The consumption of mutton is three times greater in managerial families than in labourer families and veal consumption is two times greater. Disparities between social classes are equally large for certain fresh vegetables and fruits. It is especially interesting to note that 'consumption models' are clearly different between labourers and clerical workers although the incomes of these two salary catagories are similar. Clerical workers (as compared to labourers) eat less bread, less sausage products and in general less pork, but more chicken and fish, notably less sugar, and finally fewer fats.

Studies by *Pequignot* [19, 20] show that since 1972 the share of lipids in total energy input is diminishing among managers and the professions: supposedly, these professional groups have found out, before other social categories, the risks associated with excessive lipid input.

In France as in all the industrialized countries, the growth of large stores (supermarkets and hypermarkets) has contributed greatly to modifying nutritional behaviour. First of all because we can find in these stores exotic products (for example new exotic fruits) or new processed foods (a large choice of frozen foods or preserved foods in soft packaging) but also because self service is in itself a factor for change. Let us present one example for a well-known French product, cheese: when the housewife in the small traditional store asks for a cheese, she always asks for the same ones; in contrast, in the supermarket, she chooses with her eyes and, as in France there are more than 380 different cheeses, her choice can be very large.

Some economists and nutritionists maintain that in the coming years we will all use, according to the days of the week, two different consumption models: a daily consumption and a festive consumption for holidays, for dinners among friends and for family celebrations.

But the French attach great importance to the relationship value of a meal and to conviviality [30]. Some meals are eaten very rapidly; many people, including the young, attach importance to the conversations and social exchanges that can take place during a meal.

The fast-food phenomenon in France is growing with the same characteristics as in the USA. It is a fashion and the only new elements are the bright colours of the setting and the music (often loud). Fast food has existed over the centuries both in Europe and in North Africa, in the Middle East and elsewhere. In North Africa, for centuries and centuries, little round buns split in half with three little hot sausages inside have been sold in the streets. The development of hamburgers and similar products has been parallelled by the development of 'viennoiseries' from Vienna. Pancake houses have been offering dishes which have been traditional in Brittany for centuries: a buckwheat pancake cooked with an egg, or cheese, or ham, or sardines, or with onions. Other shops offer pizzas which as we all know are traditional Ialian dishes. All this means is that in the cities of rich countries different foods are offered which are industrial preparations or regional recipes.

In France as in other countries, there are still very few studies on the evolution of the number of meals per day and the evolution of total energy input related to the development of fast food. Certain French nutritionists along with the authors of this article see no objection – quite the contrary – to their fellow citizens eating a smaller midday meal (that is to say less energy input) on condition that they acquire the habit of having a real meal before beginning their day and leaving for work as do the British or the Dutch, for example. But Europe evolves slowly and favourable diet habits travel slowly from one country to another. In France breakfast is all too often made up of a cup of coffee and a piece of buttered bread. A large educational effort is presently under way to teach the French to better spread out their meals during the day.

The prevalence of overweight and obesity as a condition is, fortunately, less common in Europe than in the USA or in Canada. It is necesary to develop the nutritional education of the totality of the population and especially of the young so that the development of new dietary habits (fast-foods, increase in the number of meals) does not result in European countries having as high a prevalence of obesity as in the USA.

The French are still suspicious of industrially prepared foods and of preserves [13]. The consumption of canned or frozen foods is clearly less than in the USA or in neighbouring European countries. As an example, the amount of canned vegetables in 1978 was 19.8 kg/person/year in France and 42.8 kg/person/year in the USA. All this is rather strange in the country of *Nicolas Appert,* and of *Charles Tellier* (who was known as 'the father of cold' for food, and who installed the first refrigeration machine on a ship in 1865 and who equipped the first refrigeration ship). The attitude of the French towards certain industrial foods in fairly illogical. However, frozen foods have met less resistance from consumers than canned foods.

Regional Diets in France

France, due to the diversity of its countryside and to the variety of its agricultural production, has shown over preceding centuries great regional differences which have given birth to different 'cuisines', which has contributed to the fame of 'French gastronomy'.

The development of modern methods of agriculture an breeding as well as the prodigious progress (as in all industrialized countries) in food tech-

Table XIV. Regional differences in butter and oil consumption, from the INSEE [15]

	North	West	Southwest	Southeast (Mediterranean region)
Butter, kg/person/year	14.3	12.6	5.7	5.2
Oil, l/person/year	10	9.1	14.4	18.5

nology, the development of transports, population movements, increasing urbanization, and finally the organization of distribution companies countrywide, have all contributed to providing food abundance and to lessening the differences between regions.

However, there are still regional dietary habits [25, 28]. In the past, there was a 'butter France' corresponding to the north of the country and an 'oil France', corresponding to the south, and especially to the southeast. This phenomenon has lessened, but the differences still exist as can be seen in the figures in table XIV. These differences are great enough to justify epidemiological studies, as those of *Renaud* [21], comparing two departments with different lipid consumptions and including biological studies on blood lipids as well as studies on aggregate blood platelets.

The Mediterranean region, in contact with Italy, has dietary habits similar to it: the consumption of olive oil, pasta, and tomatoes (all products appreciated by the Italians) are noticeably higher than in the rest of France [15, 26, 28]. The North and the East consume many more potatoes than the rest of France (60% more than the national average) and these regions have dietary habits close to their neighbours, Belgium and Germany. The same holds for beer consumption. But beer is no longer a beverage limited to the regions of the North and the East. Its use is spreading throughout France due to company restaurants where beer competes directly with wine. Cider was the traditional beverage in Brittany and other western provinces, but its use is decreasing, replaced by beer or wine.

We mentioned before the rapid increase in cheese consumption. 10 years ago (1972), the average amount consumed varied by as much as 100% according to the regions (the highest consumption being in the East, the centre and the Paris region). These differences are diminishing due to people travelling in the country, but especially due to the evolution of distribution and to advertising on television.

We are heading towards the use over the whole of the country of products and culinary specialties of all the different regions. At the same time we are welcoming foreign specialties from neighbouring countries, but also from North Africa due to the ties between this region and France and because of the presence in France of large numbers of immigrant workers from Algeria, Morocco and Tunisia. Many Vietnamese and Chinese restaurants have opened in the large cities during these last years, and Asiatic cuisine is today present (with adaptations for local taste) throughout the world.

Conclusions

In France, as in all the industrialized countries, nutritional habits have undergone a profound upheaval during the last decades. The role of different foods in the diet and the composition of this diet have profoundly changed. But nutrition is such a daily fact and so repetitive that consumers have not become fully aware of this revolution.

It would be useful if our contemporaries were better informed of the changes that have taken place in the production, the preservation, the industrial transformation and the commercialization of foods. It is to be hoped that they become better informed of the favourable consequences of the new techniques (abundance, diversity, ease of cooking, uniformity of the characteristics of industrial products, etc.) and also better informed of the new risks for public health associated with this abundance, with this facility, and with the choice that we make every day in the composition of our meals. The Commission which, under the presidency of one of the authors, published in 1981 the work *Recommended Dietary Allowances for the French Population* [8] mentioned briefly in the opening pages of this work the evolution in life and work styles and the evolution of diet.

Epidemiological studies of the relationship between diet and health (or diet and pathology) can only be carried out successfully by multidisciplinary research groups [4, 10] and call for much caution in interpreting the facts. Those researchers interested in nutrition or epidemiology or in public health need to know not only the present diet of the human group or peoples that they are studying, but also the transformations in that diet during the 40–50 preceding years. We therefore feel it is useful to collect detailed and precise data on the evolution of nutrition in one country, France, and to briefly give certain elements of comparison with other countries.

References

1 Aron, J.P.: Le mangeur du XIXe siècle (Laffont, Paris 1973).

2 Claudian, J.; Serville, Y.: Evolution récente des coutumes alimentaires en France. Cah. Nutr. Diét. *5:* 41–53 (1970).

3 Combris, P.: Les grands traits de l'évolution de la consommation alimentaire en France de 1956 à 1976. C.r. Acad. Agric. Fr *15:* 1273–1284 (1980).

4 Debry, G.: Nutrition de santé publique: illusions ou réalités? Cah. Nutr. Diét. *9:* 15–26 (1974).

5 Ducimetière, P.: Cardiopathies ischémiques: incidences comparées en France, en Europe et aux Etats-Unis. Concours méd. *103:* 6463–6469 (1981).

6 Ducimetière, P.: Etudes comparées dans le monde de la fréquence de l'athérosclérose. Revue Pratn *29:* 603–614 (1979).

7 Dupin, H.: L'alimentation des Français, évolution et problèmes nutritionnels (ESF, Paris 1978).

8 Dupin, H. et Commission du CNERNA: Apports nutritionnels conseillés pour la population française (Techniques et Documentation Lavoisier, Paris 1981).

9 FAO (Food and Agriculture Organization): Bilans alimentaires moyens 1975–1977 et disponibilités alimentaires par personne (moyennes 1961–65, 1967 à 1977) (FAO, Roma 1980).

10 Fauconneau, G.: La recherche en matière d'agro-industries en France. Revue Synth. *1977:* 76–87.

11 Feron, R.: Consommation lipidique des Français de 1965 a 1974. Ann. Nutr. Aliment. *30:* 141–160 (1976).

12 Feron, R.: Consommation lipidique des Français de 1974 à 1980 (personal communication).

13 Fondation Française pour la Nutrition: Les Français et leur alimentation (FFN, Paris 1978).

14 Grignon, C.; Grignon, C.: Alimentation et stratification sociale. Cah. Nutr. Diét. *16:* 207–217 (1981).

15 Mercier, M.A.: La consommation alimentaire en 1977. Les collections de l'INSEE. Série M, No. 83 (INSEE, Paris 1980).

16a Bilans alimentaires et autres bilans; rétrospectives 1959–1974. Collection des statistiques agricoles. Etude No. 139 (Ministère de l'Agriculture. Service Central des Enquêtes et Etudes Statistiques, Paris 1975).

16b Résultats 1975–76–77. Collection des statistiques agricoles, publié en 1978. Résultats 1977–78, publié en 1979. Résultats 1980, publié en 1981 (Ministère de l'Agriculture. Service Central des Enquêtes et Etudes Statistiques, Paris).

17 Niaudet, J.: Les dépenses des Français pour leur alimentation. Annls Nutr. Aliment. *30:* 429–437 (1976).

18 OCDE (Organisation de Coopération et de Développement Economique): Statistiques de consommation des denrées alimentaires (OECD Food Consumption Statistics.) (OCDE, Paris 1981).

19 Pequignot, G.: La consommation alimentaire des adultes en France. Annls Nutr. Aliment. *30:* 175–184 (1976).

20 Pequignot, G.: La consommation alimentaire des Français en fonction de la taille des

agglomérations, reflet de l'évolution longitudinale. Revue Epidem. Santé Publ. *28:* 169–183 (1980).
21 Renaud, S.: Dietary fats and thrombosis. Biblthеca Nutr. Dieta, No. 25, pp. 92–99 (Karger, Basel 1975).
22 Richard, J.L.: Lipides alimentaires, cholestérolémie et cardiopathies ischémiques. Revue Epidem. Santé Publ. *28:* 461–484 (1980).
23 Rolland, M.F.; Chabert, J.; Serville, Y.: La consommation de pain et de ses substituts. Annls Nutr. Aliment. *31:* 105–118, 365–380 (1977).
24 Saunier, P.: Les déterminants économiques et sociaux de la nourriture dans le long terme; l'alimentation des familles ouvrières urbaines. Annls Nutr. Aliment. *30:* 439–446 (1976).
25 Serville, Y.; Guilloud-Bataille, M.: La subsistance des styles alimentaires régionaux. Ethnol. fr. *10:* 326–334 (1980).
26 Thi-Nguyen-Huu; Vengrevelingue, G.: Premiers résultats d'une enquête permanente sur la consommation alimentaire des Français. Etudes et conjoncture, No. 7, pp. 1–90 (INSEE, Paris 1967).
27 Thi-Nguyen-Huu; Richard, D.: Principaux résultats de l'enquête permanente sur la consommation alimentaire des Français. Etudes et conjoncture, No. 10, pp. 83–154 (INSEE, Paris 1968).
28 Thouvenot, C.; Favier, A.: Une méthode de cartographie de la sensibilité alimentaire en France. Ethnol. fr. *10:* 273–296 (1980).
29 Toutain, J.C.: La consommation alimentaire en France de 1789 à 1964. Cahiers de l'ISEA, Economie et Sociétés, tome V, No. 2 (Droz, Genève 1971).
30 Tremolières, J.: Diététique et art de vivre (Seghers, Paris 1975).
31 Tuyns, A.J.: Le cancer de l'œsophage en Ille et Vilaine en fonction des niveaux de consommation d'alcool et de tabac. Bull. Cancer *64:* 45–60 (1977).
32 Villeneuve, A.: Enquête permanente sur la consommation alimentaire des Français, année 1972. Les collections de l'INSEE, série M, No. 34 (INSEE, Paris 1974).

H. Dupin, MD, Institut Scientifique et Technique de l'Alimentation, CNAM, 292, rue Saint-Martin, F-75141 Paris Cedex 03 (France)

Wld Rev. Nutr. Diet., vol. 44, pp. 85–116 (Karger, Basel 1984)

Thiamin – the Interaction of Aging, Alcoholism, and Malabsorption in Various Populations

Richard A. Baum, Frank L. Iber

University of Maryland School of Medicine, Division of Gastroenterology, and Baltimore VA Medical Center, Baltimore, Md., USA

Contents

This review is based upon data that is highly incomplete in many third world countries. It is, however, possible to look at trends with aging from the Western World of Europe and North America and make reasonable projections as to what to expect in other areas.

Thiamin (also called vitamin B_1) was among the first vitamins to have its structure identified [40, 146], its role in carbohydrate metabolism clarified [138], and effective methods of assay in urine and food developed [63].

Table I. Dietary intakes of thiamin and calories (males)

N HANES I				N HANES II			
age years	kcal	thiamin (SD)	mg/ 1,000 kcal	age years	kcal	thiamin (SD)	mg/ 1,000 kcal
1–74	2,393	1.52 (0.59)	0.64	0.5–74	2,381	1.56 (1.06)	0.65
25–34	2,793	1.60 (0.62)	0.62	25–34	2,734	1.69 (1.18)	0.62
35–44	2,554	1.55 (0.59)	0.61	35–44	2,424	1.55 (1.20)	0.64
45–54	2,301	1.47 (0.61)	0.64	45–54	2,361	1.51 (0.85)	0.64
55–64	2,076	1.40 (0.52)	0.68	55–64	2,071	1.40 (0.79)	0.68
65–74	1,805	1.38 (0.48)	0.77	65–74	1,828	1.33 (0.88)	0.73

Table II. Dietary intakes of thiamin and calories (females)

N HANES I				N HANES II			
age years	kcal	thiamin (SD)	mg/ 1,000 kcal	age years	kcal	thiamin (SD)	mg/ 1,000 kcal
1–74	1,618	1.12 (0.56)	0.69	0.5–74	1,578	1.06 (0.72)	0.68
25–34	1,638	1.08 (0.48)	0.66	25–34	1,643	1.08 (0.90)	0.66
35–44	1,558	1.04 (0.37)	0.67	35–44	1,579	1.05 (0.83)	0.66
45–54	1,533	1.07 (0.44)	0.70	45–54	1,439	0.98 (0.58)	0.68
55–64	1,382	1.02 (0.31)	0.74	55–64	1,401	1.00 (0.62)	0.71
65–74	1,307	1.00 (0.39)	0.77	65–74	1,295	0.99 (0.76)	0.76

Thiamin requirements in humans were established by the mid-1940s [50, 106, 143, 144] and a close relationship between thiamin requirements and total caloric intake was noted. Thiamin deficiency develops in people whose diets contain less than 0.2 mg/day. After several weeks of such a diet, loss of appetite and inanition occur followed after several months by cardiovascular and neurological changes.

Thiamin is widely available in the diet of North Americans. The mandatory enrichment of flour with thiamin in the USA as well as enrichment of other foods and availability of vitamin supplements have virtually eliminated clinical thiamin deficiency in North America except in conditions which interfere with ingestion or absorption of food for long periods of time. Alcoholism is the cardinal example of such a condition but other chronic illnesses can also produce thiamin deficiency.

In the tropics subclinical intestinal damage usually discussed under the title of tropical sprue is widely prevalent and increases the need for dietary thiamin for it is not adequately absorbed. Flour enrichment programs do not exist.

I. Thiamin Intake

Thiamin intake is adequate in the world except when there is starvation, or polished rice is the main dietary constituent [74, 103–105].

The most extensive information on thiamin intake in the USA is found in two surveys conducted by the National Health and Nutrition Surveys – N HANES I (1971–74) [1] and N HANES II (1976–80) [39]. These surveys were conducted by the National Center for Health Statistics, US Department of Health and Human Services. Data were gathered from a cross-sectional sample of the United States civilian non-institutionalized population.

A 24-hour recall method was employed to develop intake data. Physical health of respondents was determined by questionnaire and data was obtained on many specific dietary items. Tables I and II present data from these studies on both caloric and thiamin intake in patients aged 25–74 grouped by decade cohorts. Data was not obtained in patients older than 74 years.

These data indicate that at all ages Americans are, on the average, ingesting thiamin in excess of 0.6 mg/1,000 cal. In young men [117], diets containing 0.3 mg/1,000 cal do not produce biochemical evidence of thia-

Table III. Intake of calories and thiamin

Region	Sex	a	Age mean or range	kcal mean/ 24 h	mg thiamin, kcal		Comment
Boston [89]	M	31	M 65	2,458	1.3	0.52	free-living
	F	69	M 65	1,831	0.94	0.51	
Nebraska [58]	M	11	58–83	1,812	1.2	0.66	congregate meals
	F	19	58–83	1,475	0.9	0.61	
Vancouver [85]	M	74	M 77	1,867	1.0	0.53	singles or couples
	F	76	M 74	1,449	0.9	0.62	
Oregon [147]	M	23	M 74	2,177	1.3	0.62	free-living
	F	75	M 74	1,586	1.2	0.69	
Indiana [77]	M	12	63–93	1,609	1.1	0.69	private nursing home
	F	32	63–93	1,388	0.9	0.65	
Colorado [122]	M	23	62–98	1,720	1.0	0.60	nursing home
	F	23	62–98	1,333	0.67	0.50	ambulatory
Colorado [60]	F	24	62–99	1,381	1.2	0.87	free-living

min deficiency. Although caloric intake decreases with age, the calorie-corrected thiamin intake does not. In lower socioeconomic groups ingestion of food and thiamin is also decreased but even in these groups N HANES II data reveals thiamin intake in excess of 0.5 mg/1,000 cal. Older people and poorer people, as noted in N HANES II, consumed less meat and more cereal than the younger, more affluent segment of society. Frequently, however, cereals are enriched with thiamin and thus compensate for decreased meat intake. This does not apply to the rest of the world where cereals are not enriched.

Smaller surveys of thiamin intake are available in a number of well-defined populations. Table III summarizes studies on healthy ambulatory older Americans and indicates adequate thiamin intake in free living and in uninstitutionalized persons. *Justice* et al. [77] observed food intake on 5 nonconsecutive days by elderly patients in a private nursing home. The population was subdivided into 23 patients under 84 and 21 over. There was no significant difference in thiamin intake between these two groups. *Steidemann* et al. [122] weighed the food intake on 3 successive days on ambulatory nursing home patients. They too compared calorie and thiamin intake of persons aged 60–84 and 85–95. Ingested calories fell in the older group but thiamin intake per 1,000 cal was essentially unchanged (0.54 mg/1,000 cal in the younger group, 0.5 mg/1,000 cal in the older). It is noteworthy that in this study people with free access to diets prepared with RDA amounts of food and specific nutrients ate less than the single day estimates of N HANES I and N HANES II, and less than the RDA.

An important European study by *Vir and Love* [135] was done in Belfast and examined weighed intake of food on three consecutive days by 196 subjects who could be grouped by living conditions as: (1) institutionalized in hospitals; (2) living in sheltered dwellings; (3) residential accommodations with meals provided; (4) free-living. Little difference was found in thiamin intake as related to calorie intake in various living conditions ranging from 0.39 to 0.46 mg thiamin/1,000 cal/day.

The observed intake of thiamin in this study is about one third lower than that of N HANES II and is in the range of the lowest intakes observed in that study. When the thiamin status of the Belfast population was evaluated by transketolase assay, however, there was marked variation in status from subgroup to subgroup despite similar intakes. Thus, in one hospital only 1 of 54 patients was marginally thiamin-deficient by transketolase assay while another 10 of 43 were either marginally or severely deficient. 7 of 20 people in a sheltered dwelling and 6 of 53 free-living people showed marginally deficient thiamin status. Intakes in this study were substantially less than in the USA but it clearly demonstrates that thiamin deficiency by biochemical criteria can develop at lower intakes.

It is clear from the available data that for all American population groups thiamin intake is above 0.5 mg/1,000 cal and is thus able to prevent thiamin deficiency. Individuals eating less than this amount in a healthy free-living population are quite uncommon.

Thiamin availability in the diet in other portions of the world has been widely surveyed. Apart from starvation and regions predominantly dependent upon polished rice, it is clear that marginal thiamin intakes are usually found in the poorest group of subjects and the elderly may well be included. Thus, surveys continue to demonstrate beriberi in Ethiopia, the Sudan, Mozambique, Nigeria, and Gabon in significant numbers of cases indicating thiamin deficiency [93–95].

II. Thiamin Absorption

Thiamin is absorbed by two distinct mechanisms best demonstrated in rats by *Hoyumpa* et al. [69, 70]. The first mechanism of absorption is active, the second passive. The active mechanism requires oxygen and energy and is capable of transporting thiamin against a concentration gradient. At intestinal concentrations of thiamin above 3 μ*M*, the active transport mechanism is saturated and passive absorption takes place. It is estimated that in man consuming 2.0 mg daily of thiamin or less that the concentration in the intestinal lumen will be usually less than 2 μ*M* but there are no direct measurements of luminal thiamin concentrations in man nor is there specific information on how thiamin is absorbed.

Indirect measurement of thiamin absorption has been made in man after single oral doses of 1.0–50.0 mg. Many of these data in man show no well-defined dose-related absorptive differences consistent with simple passive transport [7, 55, 69, 96] but some studies show saturation kinetics [38, 127, 136]. The study of the absorption of thiamin HCl in one dose under these circumstances is not the same as thiamin consumed as part of a meal and the indirect techniques used to assess absorption do not provide clear understanding of dietary thiamin absorption in man. There are no adequate studies of thiamin absorption with aging. In young adults free of alcoholism data suggest that absorption is complete [127, 128]. With aging, small intestinal villus surface diminishes [139] and the amount of digestive enzyme per unit weight of mucosa falls [66]. However, this is generally compensated for by the reserve capacity of the small intestine and malabsorption as a biological function of aging remains at a level far below the clinical threshold.

The intestinal absorptive function in normal subjects living in tropical areas is not the same as those in temperate climates. The mucosal biopsy shows changes of flattening that seem due to a combination of bacterial overgrowth and folic acid deficiency. This lesion interferes measurably with the active transport of most absorptive processes and there is every reason to believe that such interference is also present for thiamin. It is our view that the magnitude of the interference is about the same as that of alcoholism in North America, thus the marginally sufficient diets with the presence of a small intestine lesion is converted to a severe deficiency through the inability to absorb the thiamin [80, 86–88].

Impairment of thiamin absorption has been demonstrated primarily in alcoholism. *Thomson* and co-workers [124, 126, 127] demonstrated inhibition of thiamin absorption: (a) in malnourished alcoholics with and without liver disease, (b) in healthy volunteers who were administered 1.5 g/kg of ethanol prior to a single dose of thiamin. In the alcoholic group thiamin absorption reverted to normal after 6 weeks of abstinence from alcohol. The alcoholics in this study had other signs and symptoms of malabsorption but the volunteer subjects did not. *Tomasulo* et al. [128] demonstrated malabsorption of thiamin in alcoholics free of liver disease and return to normal with correction of malnutrition. This was one of many abnormalities in absorption that became normal after 14 days of abstinence and nutritional repletion. Malabsorption of thiamin was postulated to be related to an alcohol induced injury to the small intestinal mucosa. Thiamin deficiency as detected by biochemical tests is present in 25% of alcoholics admitted to general hospitals in the USA [82, 83]. A representative survey is reported recently on 50 chronic alcoholics seen at the medical emergency ward of the Basle University Hospital with alcohol-related illness who were examined by the transketolase activation effect of thiamin pyrophosphate (TPP). 23 of this group (46%) were abnormal in comparison to only 2% of 1,152 healthy adult controls [62].

The data of *Thomson* and co-workers [125, 127] make it clear that the amont of alcohol in two portions of beer, wine, or whiskey is sufficient to interfere with thiamin absorption as a single dose. It requires continuous drinking, however, to block the majority of thiamin absorption and produce thiamin deficiency.

The N HANES II included alcoholic beverages in its surveys of food intake and found that average intake peaked in the 4th and 5th decades and then tapered off. Men drink more than women and alcohol provides 5–6% of daily calories. This data thus indicates that alcohol use is prevalent but provides no information on the incidence of alcoholism or whether prevalent alcohol use impacts on thiamin absorption.

Data on alcoholism in the elderly is limited. 9% of all Americans over the age of 18 are estimated to be alcoholics. It is generally accepted that males in the 4th and 5th decades have the highest incidence. Evaluation of recently admitted patients to public wards or public nursing homes indicates 15–20% are chronic alcoholics [79, 118]. Of patients over the age of 60, 2–10% are estimated to be alcoholics [149] and the percentage is thought to be higher in those in nursing homes. Loss of physical and mental ability, loss of dentition and bereavement are all thought to contribute to increased alcohol use among the elderly and alcoholism in the older population is recognized as being underdiagnosed.

Hoyumpa et al. [69] extended studies of alcohol and thiamin to evaluate the mechanism of inhibition of absorption of the latter by the former. Modest doses of alcohol (50 mg/100 g body weight) given intragastrically or intravenously interfered with thiamin absorption at the low concentrations associated with active transport. Analysis of this interference indicated that the uptake of thiamin from the intestinal lumen was normal but that the egress of thiamin from the mucosal cell was blocked by alcohol. This blockage was caused by ethanol interference with a NaK ATPase. Similar results were found with ouabain.

The impairment of absorption found in alcoholism has many similarities to the changes found in absorption in tropical or third world persons. The lesion in the tropics is more advanced, in that there is usually a biopsy abnormality but the broad interference with absorption of actively transported substances is quite similar [80, 86–88]. The most severe and best studied form of this disease is found under the heading tropical sprue, but most systematic studies indicate that this disease is but an extreme form of changes that in lesser degree are regarded as normal [100]. The extensive occurrence of folate deficiency in these persons in the presence of diets adequate in folate suggest wide impairment of B vitamin absorption. This condition, much more prevalent in the world than alcoholism, would be expected to contribute in a major way to the finding of thiamin impairment in tropical populations and combined with impaired intakes makes thiamin deficiency prominent in surveys.

No data has been located on increases in this intestinal lesion with aging. The lesion seems of multifactorial origin including impaired protein intake as well characterized in kwashiorkor, folate deficiency, giardia and bacterial overgrowth, and helminth infestations. Only protein deficiency would be anticipated to worsen as the subjects become older.

Alcohol can thus be concluded to be the most important factor in the bioavailability of thiamin as an American population. In all American series of Wernicke-Korsakoff disease – the most specific of the thiamin deficiency states – nearly all cases arise in alcoholic patients. Heavy intake of alcohol interferes with gut function in a broad manner [98]. Alcohol also affects intermediary metabolism of thiamin-increasing requirement [52, 82].

Possible interference with thiamin absorption by coffee is reported by *Somogyi and Nageli* [120]. 25 young volunteers were given 7 cups of coffee versus an equal amount of water and then had urinary thiamin excretion measured after a test dose. Urinary excretion was 45% less in the subjects receiving coffee.

Some indigenous habits seem to contribute to thiamin deficiency. It has been demonstrated that tea leaves [64, 134], betel nuts [133], and fermented fish [133] interfere with thiamin availability, even when the diet is adequate. *Vimokesant* et al. [133] showed that 10 of 30 Thai subjects had a deficient TPP stimulation effect on their erythrocytes while they were using betel nuts and eating fermented fish. All but 1 of these were restored to normal by dropping both habits.

III. Biochemical Pathways Status

Thiamin exists in food in water-soluble forms, mostly as free thiamin or as phosphate esters which are hydrolyzed in the lumen of the small intestine to the free form. Lipid soluble forms of thiamin have been made synthetically and are absorbed in the same manner as long chain fatty acids through the lymphatics. *Thomson* et al. [126] investigated the effectiveness of these lipid soluble forms (allithiamin) using thiamin propyldisulfide and thiamin tetrahydrofurfuryl disulfide. Both of these compounds were capable of restoring blood, urine, and red cell thiamin parameters to normal in alcoholics [136]. Experience with these synthetic thiamin conjugates is limited and as yet they have no clear role in therapy [17, 126, 136].

Upon absorption free thiamin is phosphorylated in the intestinal epithelial cell and enters the blood almost entirely as the pyrophosphate ester

[112]. Many tissues besides the intestine can phosphorylate thiamin while the liver is capable of thiamin storage [145].

TPP acts as a cofactor in several enzyme systems essential to the function of nearly all cells including neurons and glia. Thiamin also plays a direct role in the excitability of neurons [75, 148]. In normal animals, the heart, kidney, liver, and brain have the highest thiamin concentration [61]. Substantially smaller amounts are found in spleen, lung, adrenal and muscle. Subcellular distribution of thiamin as detected by radiolabelled techniques reveals 60–70% in the mitochondria with about 20% of its total thiamin in microsomes compared to only 8% in liver and kidney [18]. There is no information on the effect of aging on thiamin distribution in man or animals.

IV. Determination of Thiamin Status

Determination of thiamin status has been made by direct measurement of blood levels of thiamin or TPP. Thiamin stores have been indirectly measured by the urinary excretion of thiamin and its metabolites. Thiamin state of tissues has been measured by assay of thiamin-dependent enzymes especially in red cells (transketolase) and white cells. The stimulatory effect of added TPP on enzyme activity has also been measured.

Blood levels of thiamin and TPP are indirect measures of tissue stores compared to direct measurement of tissue levels but in some animals studies they have been quite sensitive [14, 19, 61]. In depletion states, the excretion of intact thiamin in the urine drops nearly to zero before tissue stores are diminished. Blood and muscle levels in man parallel depletion [102].

In rodents given oral-labelled thiamin, the excretion in the urine accounts for 90% of the administered dose in replete animals [97, 129]. The major urinary products are free thiamin and thiazole rings with different side groups, in total about 20 different metabolites have been identified [19, 102].

Thiamin turnover seems accelerated in deficient animals [19] and the level of intake of thiamin clearly determines both the amount and chemical form of urinary excretion. The turnover has been reported in 2 normal men and the estimated biological half-life was 18 and 24 days [13] while a depleted person had a turnover of 6 days [14]. The more rapid turnover with depletion and the ability to produce depletion in as little as 14 days seems best explained by a diminished distribution in the depleted state.

TPP is the active coenzyme form of thiamin and it functions in a variety of simple or oxidative decarboxylations of pyruvic acids and ketoglutaric acid and branch chain alpha beta acids. The studies of *Rindi and DeGiuseppe* [111] have made it possible to measure monophosphoric and triphosphoric esters of thiamin as well as TPP. *Airth and Foerster* [4] have adapted these methods to whole blood.

The assessment of thiamin status improved markedly when in 1953 it was discovered that one of the enzymes of the hexose monophosphate shunt (transketolase) present in red cells required TPP as a cofactor [68, 110]. *Brin* [30] and *Brin* et al. [33, 34] are largely responsible for the establishment of the assay of this enzyme in erythrocytes as the most practical method for determining an individual's thiamin status. Transketolase activity in blood in most cases is a good reflection of thiamin nutrition as best demonstrated in Wernicke-Korsakoff syndrome where transketolase activity is invariably depressed [45]. Magnesium deficiency also affects transketolase activity, however, and transketolase activity thus may not accurately recommend thiamin status in hypomagnesemic individuals [49].

Other TPP-dependent enzymes have also been evaluated as indices of thiamin nutrition. These include the ketoglutarate dehydrogenase complex, the pyruvate dehydrogenase complex, and the branched chain dehydrogenase complex [26, 45, 49]. All of these enzyme systems are present in white cells or fibroblasts and their activities can be measured by incubating white cells or fibroblasts with the appropriate radiolabelled substrate and measuring the radioactive carbon dioxide that evolves. Activity can be stimulated by adding TPP to the reaction mixture [25, 47]. These assays, however, are not well standardized and vary markedly with small changes in technique [46, 81].

A substantial body of evidence indicates that thiamin and probably its triphosphate ester play an important role in membrane function perhaps related to sodium channels [22, 44]. Attempts have been made to evaluate this function clinically most notably by tests for a putative 'inhibitor' of thiamin triphosphate [43, 108]. However, the normal assay for the inhibitor does not use the membrane bound physiological substrate required to show net synthesis of thiamin triphosphate [116], indicating that improved clinically clarified assays are needed.

Difficulties in measuring thiamin directly were largely overcome by the introduction of the thiochrome urinary method [107]. This highly fluorescent molecule is relatively stable and results from both free thiamin and several of its metabolites giving values which are always higher than a true thiamin assay on the same urine [117]. A variety of thiamin requiring organisms including *Lactobacillus viridescens* [117] and *Ochromonas danica* [15] have been used. Both are more specific and much more sensitive than the thiochrome assay but also detect some metabolite. High performance liquid chromatography is quite capable now of detecting thiamin and its metabolites [76] in urine even in depleted subjects and can be also applied to blood measurements.

Sauberlich et al. [117] investigated the clinical and biochemical changes in 7 young men maintained on thiamin-deficient diets of varying caloric content. The urinary assay of excreted thiamin by both *L. viridescens* and thiochrome methods indicated a clear fall in the first few days. In this manner, on a very low thiamin intake, the urinary thiamin excretion by the *L. viridescens* method fell from a mean of over 100 mg/24 h to less than 25 mg/24 h and reached depleted levels by the 14th day. Although the fall in level of excretion and the diagnosis of depletion was equally identified by the thiochrome method, it was not nearly as sensitive. The *L. viridescens* assay responded to some molecules other than the parent one [10]. Both this assay and the *O. danica* one used by *Baker* seem similarly useful. *Ziporin* et al. [150] noted that the thiamin-depleted individual has more pyrimidine and thiazole metabolites of thiamin.

Thus, all of the methods used in the survey of urine seem to lack specificity for thiamin. Catabolism of thiamin continues and perhaps increases with depletion. The nearer a method directly measures thiamin alone the better it serves as a survey tool. The microbiological methods approach this ideal far more closely than thiochrome but an improved method is desirable. At present, the protozoological method (with *O. danica*) and the bacteriological one (with *L. viridescens*) seem to reflect most clearly thiamin levels and to be last influenced by catabolic products. The sensitivity, specificity and reliability in the detection and monitoring of thiamin depletion is not unlimited by any of these methods, however.

The erythrocyte transketolase activity has been widely studied and many descriptions of methods have appeared indicating problems with standardization. The most widely employed method of quantitating a thiamin effect is to determine the percentage increase in the reaction rate produced by the addition of optimal amounts of TPP to the reaction mixture – the TPP effect. In the *Sauberlich* et al. [117] study of young persons, it was clear that levels of thiamin of 0.3 mg/1,000 kcal were required to

Table IV. Blood and urine measurements of thiamin status

Method	Reference	Severely depleted	Marginally	Adequate
Blood thiamin, ng/ml				
protozological *(O. danica)*	84	<20	20–25	20–70
	16	<20	20–25	>25
Urine thiamin thiochrome				
µg/g creatinine	107	<38	38–115	>115
µg/24 h		<38	38–200	>200
Urine-microbiological				
(L. viridescens), µg/24 h	117	<50	50–75	>75
Blood transketolase				
(red blood cells) % TPP effect	31	>25	15–24	0–14

restore urinary excretion of thiamin to normal levels or to restore erythrocyte transketolase activity to normal. Absolute transketolase levels or the TPP effect were equally sensitive indicators of thiamin status in this study.

Baker et al. [16] recently used the *O. danica* assay of whole blood to determine thiamin and TPP blood levels of 204 subjects aged 20–50 and compared them with a group of elderly patients. These authors have found excellent correlation between this microbiological protozoan assay and direct measure of muscle or liver thiamin stores in a few patients.

A variety of papers exist in which erythrocyte transketolase and blood or urine thiamin is measured. In general, correlation is good for depleted patients but some discrepancies have been noted [12, 16, 20, 35, 84]. Table IV lists reasonable criteria for considering a patient thiamin depleted by biochemical or microbiological criteria.

V. Thiamin Status of Older Americans

The thiamin status of older North Americans and Europeans is presented in table V. In general, the data indicate that deficiency of thiamin and its phosphate ester coenzyme forms is not common among free-living older people in the USA. Data from Ireland [135], the Netherlands [67], and the United Kingdom [59], where thiamin intakes are comparable to the

Table V. Thiamin status in the elderly

Reference	n	Age, mean or range	Site	Living status	Method	Fraction-deficient		
						severe %	marginal %	adequate %
16	327	60–83	Maryland	nursing home	blood thiamin	?	11	89
16	146	60–83	Virginia	free-living	blood thiamin	10	15	75
31	234	70	New York State	free-living	TPP effect[1]	3	17	80
31	45	68		VA Hospital	TPP effect	7	31	62
32	10	62–96	New York State	nursing home ill	TPP effect	10	30	60
					urine thiochrome	50	50	
60	70	62–99	Colorado	home and nursing home	urine thiochrome	37	14	73
122	46	62–98	Colorado	nursing home	urine thiochrome		19	71
85	150	>65	Vancouver	free-living	urine thiochrome			100
135	97	65–94	Belfast	geriatric hospital		1	11	88
135	46	65–95	Belfast	nursing home	TPP effect	2	19	79
135	53	65–91	Belfast	free-living			12	88
59	118	81	England	free-living	TPP effect	15	53	32
114	75	72	Helsinki	old age home	TPP effect		45	55
67	153	65–93	Netherlands	hospital	TPP effect	6	25	69

[1] TPP effect is percentage increase in transketolase activity with addition of TPP.

lower among Americans (N HANES II) [39], indicate an increasing occurrence of marginal or severe deficiency with age. The studies of *Markkanen* et al. [92] from Finland found that older persons had lower levels of erythrocyte transketolase than younger individuals. Their study was based on 414 individuals judged to be normal and in good nutritional status. The age range was newborn to 90 years. Regression analysis showed a mild decline with age but all of the factors of food availability and possible alcoholism could not be fully controlled.

In North America there is an increase among the infirm in patients showing marginal to severe thiamin deficiency. Disease seems clearly to increase the frequency and severity of deficiency. We can conclude that deficiency of thiamin and its phosphate ester coenzymes is present in about 10% of the older persons in the USA. The large surveys of *Baker* et al. [16] and *Brin* et al. [31] are the most convincing. *Baker* et al. [16, 17] using the *O. danica* assay demonstrated that 11% of 452 Americans, age 60–83, had blood levels more than 2 SD below the mean for 204 younger persons aged 20–50. *Brin* et al. [31] found approximately 20% of their 279 New York State residents had diminished urinary excretion of thiamin while a lower percentage had severe deficiency as measured by the TPP effect on the erythrocyte transketolase activity. An even higher percentage had marginal deficiency by this method.

A more pertinent question than thiamin status is adequacy of thiamin-dependent function. Functionally significant deficit of TPP or its dependent enzyme systems is more likely to be clinically manifest. Significant evidence exists for functional deficiency due to inadequate saturation with TPP in a significant subgroup of older people, particularly those who are chronically ill in the USA and Northern European societies (table V). *Brin* et al. [31] found only 0–3% of 234 volunteers ranging in age from their mid-40s to their mid-90s had abnormal TPP effect on transketolase but the proportion rose to 7% in a Veterans Hospital. *Vir and Love* [135] found an excess TPP effect on transketolase from 15 to 18% of geriatric outpatients and *Hoorn* et al. [67] found an even higher incidence of excess transketolase effect in a municipal hospital in New Jersey serving a relatively poor population.

The question of malabsorption of thiamin needs consideration in an older population. *Baker* et al. [16] reported patients with low levels of blood thiamin who were taking vitamin supplements in the hospital. *Leevy* et al. [83] studied this malabsorption in alcoholics of younger ages and showed quite clearly that there was a major impairment from alcohol effects. *Thomson and Leevy* [127] have studied a patient with surgical resection of the small bowel who did not absorb thiamin normally. Alcoholism and extensive disease or resection of small intestine seem the only causes for thiamin malabsorption, however. Generally absorption of thiamin is satisfactory as demonstrated by the fact that clinical syndromes of thiamin deficiency respond readily to oral therapy.

Blass and Gibson [27, 28] have put forth evidence that a genetic variation in thiamin-dependent enzymes may be an important factor in the clinical manifestation of thiamin deficiency by impairing the ability to utilize marginal amounts of vitamins. These workers cultured fibroblasts from 4 patients with Wernicke-Korsakoff syndrome and many control subjects and determined that the binding of TPP was 12-fold higher for the Wernicke-Korsakoff-derived fibroblasts than for controls. This binding difference persisted through several passages through tissue culture. Inherent and presumably genetic variations in thiamin binding have been described for transketolase [27, 28] as well as the other TPP-dependent enzymes [24, 46, 47, 141] each in a few individuals with relatively severe neurological disease. Mild variations might occur on the basis of genetic heterogenicity and become functionally significant in older people with marginal thiamin intake or absorption. This is an area which requires further investigation. Those few individuals who maintain a persistent abnormality of an enzymatic index of thiamin nutriture despite adequate oral repletion with vitamins should particularly be studied.

VI. Thiamin Deficiency – Animal Experience

Cardiac and CNS lesions analogous to those in man can be readily produced in experimental animals. Animal studies are difficult to interpret because severe anorexia accompanies thiamin deficiency. Inanition control animals (pair fed) are usually adequate [54]. It is clear that cardiac lesions similar to those in man have been produced in rats, dogs, cats, swine, and monkeys. CNS lesions have been produced in many species but the lesions differ in distribution from one species to another. Overall neurological lesions resemble those found in human Wernicke-Korsakoff disease.

The effects of thiamin depletion on the peripheral nervous system are less clear in experimental animals [131]. The majority of adequately controlled studies have failed to show peripheral nerve lesions which could not be accounted for by inanition. Although healing of nerves is impaired [48, 51], an exemplary experiment in thiamin-deficient Rhesus monkeys [113] failed to show peripheral nerve damage at a time when CNS damage was advanced.

A recent review paper by *Gibson* et al. [57] outlines the variety of animal behavior abnormalities found in thiamin deficiency. Herein the authors develop the view that the metabolism of neurotransmitters including acetylcholine, serotonin and amino acids is impaired in thiamin deficiency and may account for many symptoms. In animals, they review data showing impaired maze learning, avoidance conditioning and abnormal complex neurological coordinators associated with thiamin deficiency. *Plaitakis* et al. [109] have reviewed data on altered brain neurotransmitter systems in thiamin deficiency.

In man, thiamin deficiency has produced anorexia, irritability and weight loss. Electrocardiographic alteration has been produced [140, 143] as well as numbness of the toes consistent with peripheral nerve involvement [142, 143]. Documentation of clear advanced peripheral nerve injury in man has not occurred [101, 144].

VII. Clinical Manifestations of Thiamin Depletion

The term beriberi is derived from the Singhalese word beri meaning weakness and refers to the clinical spectrum of thiamin deficiency. Classically, there are two major types – dry beriberi in which the features of peripheral neuropathy are predominant and wet beriberi where the signs and symptoms of high output cardiac failure dominate. In reality clinical beriberi is usually a mixed deficiency syndrome which seems to be totally absent in populations which eat adequate thiamin (0.3 mg/1,000 kcal). These populations, of course, almost invariably have adequate intake of other B vitamins.

The diagnostic criteria for cardiac beriberi have been clearly elucidated by *Blankenhorn* [71]: (1) absence of other etiologic factors, (2) history of at least three months of gross dietary thiamin deficiency, (3) simultaneous peripheral neuritis, (4) cardiomegaly with sinus rhythm, (5) edema, (6) non-specific ST-T changes that respond to thiamin within 24 h, (7) response to therapy within 48 h with symptomatic and cardiac function improvement. The last of these criteria is most important, a therapeutic trial of thiamin is unlikely to hurt anyone with heart disease of other etiology.

Clinically, the primary features of beriberi heart disease are those of biventricular failure with right-sided failure being more prominent. Sinus tachycardia, wide pulse pressure, sweating and warm skin are usual findings. In the acute fulminant form there is severe hypotension, lactic acidosis and very low peripheral resistance [5]. Low peripheral resistance is due primarily to vasodilatation in the capacitance vessels in muscle producing the effect of an arteriovenous fistula. Early in the course this low peripheral resistance is associated with signs of hyperdynamic circulation [11, 36]. Late in the course, however, as heart failure appears, cutaneous vasoconstriction occurs to maintain systemic blood pressure and the extremities become cold and cyanotic [6]. Peripheral resistance generally doubles in 12–24 h after thiamin administration.

The electrocardiogram in beriberi heart disease characteristically shows low QRS voltage, prolonged QT interval with low voltage or inversion of T waves [29]. Cardiac catheterization data indicates high cardiac index and increased consumption of oxygen with a lower ejection fraction indicating an inefficient myocardium [8, 78, 115, 121, 137].

Beriberi heart disease arises in alcoholics in present clinical experience. Because alcohol is cardiotoxic, the diagnosis is obscured and evaluation of how much cardiac dysfunction is secondary to alcohol and how much is due to thiamin deficiency is often difficult. *Ikram* et al. [73] described 5 patients among 72 alcoholics with dilated cardiomyopathy whom they felt had beriberi heart disease on the basis of their response to intravenous thiamin during cardiac catheterization (i.v. thiamin produced a fall in cardiac output) and transketolase test and concluded that this diagnosis was insufficiently appreciated.

VIII. Clinical Ramifications of Thiamin Deficiency – Neurological Disease

The characteristic CNS syndrome of thiamin deficiency is Wernicke-Korsakoff syndrome originally described in the 1880's [37, 131]. The hallmarks of this syndrome are the triad of ophthalmoplegia, ataxia and global confusion. Any one of these may be the presenting symptom. Polyneuropathy is also commonly present and was stressed by Dr. *Korsakoff* in his initial descriptions. Nystagmus is common and may be horizontal, vertical, or both. Weakness of external rectus muscles and weakness or paralysis of conjugate gaze are frequent. These syndromes arise primarily in alcoholism but may be seen in thiamin deficiency without alcoholism. Ocular abnormalities are usually corrected within minutes after intravenous thiamin providing there is no nutritional complication delaying entry of thiamin into metabolic pathways. Response is much lower in cirrhosis and is greatly delayed when there is protein or nuclei acid deficiency [41]. Both stance and gait are involved in the ataxic state and may be so marked that the subject cannot stand. In the mildest form ataxia may be manifest only in tandem walking. Ataxia improves slowly with thiamin restoration often requiring 2 weeks or more.

Mental changes occur both acutely and chronically. Acutely there is a global confusional state, typically with clouding of consciousness. Spontaneous speech is often minimal and the patient may suspend speech in mid-sentence. Disorientation especially to time and place and misidentification are common. Postural hypotension and impaired vestibular function are likewise common [23, 56]. Cerebrospinal fluid is usually normal to routine examination. Transketolase studies show an excessive TPP effect of greater than 15% with a mean of 35% in most series. Nonspecific electroencephalogrammic abnormalities also occur [53].

A chronic memory disorder – Korsakoff's psychosis – can follow the acute 'Wernicke's encephalopathy' despite vigorous treatment with thiamin. This is particularly true in cases where the acute syndrome has been unusually severe or long lasting. *Butters and Cermak* [37] have documented both the mental changes and the degree of recovery. The characteristic defect is an amnestic syndrome with profound defects in new learning and memory for recent events. Confabulation is often present but is neither invariable nor specific. Some disturbance of past memory is almost invariably found as well. Indeed, careful neuropsychiatric testing shows a variety of other deficiencies in higher integrative intellectual function. Even defects in ability to discriminate among odors has been described [90]. Patients with Korsakoff's psychosis are often so impaired as to require custodial care.

IX. Clinical Manifestations of Thiamin Deficiency – Peripheral Neuritis

The peripheral neuritis of thiamin deficiency involves both sensory and motor nerves and is symmetrical in distribution. Axonal degeneration with destruction of both the axon and the myelin sheath is seen pathologically. The most pronounced changes are observed in the longest and largest myelinated fibers. The vagus and paravertebral sympathetics may be involved in advanced cases but extensive peripheral nerve involvement is always present in such instances. In very advanced cases anterior horn and dorsal root ganglion cells show chromatolysis.

In most patients, abnormalities are found first by physical examination. Careful questioning, however, reveals symptoms of weakness, paresthesias and pain of insidious onset. The legs are almost always affected earlier and more severely than the arms. Usually motor disability predominates. Only roughly one quarter of patients indicate pain or paresthesia as the major complaint [123, 130]. Paresthesia of the legs and calves is a common complaint and the findings are invariably symmetrical. Tenderness of the muscles on pressure is common and the deep tendon reflexes in the legs are often lost out of proportion to the weakness. In the series of *Victor* et al. [131] and that of *Adams and Victor* [3] the legs were involved almost four times as often and loss of sensation alone occurred in only 5% of cases. About 40% of patients had sensory, motor and reflex loss, about 20% loss of reflexes alone, and the remainder had mixtures. The cerebral spinal fluid is nearly always normal. Recovery with treatment is slow and substantial recovery depends heavily on maintaining the muscle tone while the nerve is regenerating.

The monographs of *Butters and Cermak* [37] and that of *Victor* et al. [131] indicate the range of changed mental states and degree of recovery. There is no systematic study of how important thiamin deficiency may be in mental changes in the elderly population. Thiamin deficiency may simulate 'senile dementia' and thiamin repletion may correct the changes especially in the aged alcoholic. Clinical lesions due to thiamin deficiency are often complicated by other deficiency states so that it is necessary to also identify and correct these abnormalities [16, 17]. Rapid responsiveness to thiamin treatment establishes a cause and effect relationship between thiamin deficiency and ophthalmoplegia in Wernicke's syndrome. Similarly a dramatic decrease in cardiac output and improvement in heart function after thiamin identifies beriberi heart disease. In contrast, the slow response of peripheral neuropathy whose other nutrients may be responsible, requires biochemical confirmation.

The symptoms and signs of mild thiamin deficiency are remarkably nonspecific and are of almost no value in screening for this disease. The more advanced symptoms and signs are defined by the Wernicke-Korsakoff syndrome, peripheral neuritis or cardiomyopathy present major problems in screening the elderly. Heart disease, forgetfulness and loss of vibratory sensation in the lower extremities are quite common with aging. Peripheral neuritis has many causes. These factors in combination render the symptomatic screening for thiamin deficiency based on symptoms and physical examination of limited value in the elderly.

X. Discussion

Thiamin is an essential nutrient whose deficiency produces a variety of clinical syndromes. The best data available, however, indicates that essentially all free living Americans have diets which are adequate for thiamin. Poverty and advancing age are, however, associated with declining thiamin intakes. *Brin* et al. [31] and *Baker* et al. [16] observed impairment of biochemical thiamin status in free-living poor and those in institutions. Data from Europe [67, 114, 135] shows increasing incidence of marginal or severe thiamin depletion in elderly populations ingesting thiamin at a level of about 60% that eaten by North Americans.

The recommended daily allowance (RDA) of thiamin is 1 mg daily. This seems to be a very generous amount. Caloric intake diminished with age after age 50 by about 10% per decade. Thiamin intake is related to calorie intake and this relationship is not reflected in the RDA. There is, however, no evidence of any harmful effects from ingesting this amount.

In the face of adequate thiamin ingestion, vitamin depletion states are possible if absorption is impaired. Alcoholism is known to impair thiamin absorption and is the setting in which deficiency is most commonly seen. There are, however, no systematic investigations of alcoholism and its relation to thiamin deficiency in the elderly. Intestinal disease may also impair thiamin absorption but seem rarely implicated in thiamin deficiency. *Baker* et al. [17] observed 5 of 228 elderly nursing home residents exhibited low blood thiamin despite adequate supplementation which repleted promptly with intramuscular dosing. Others [17, 67, 135] report thiamin deficiency despite regular intake of vitamins but these data are isolated and too poorly controlled to clarify the absorption issue.

The studies of *Baker* et al. [16, 17] indicate that about 25% of the noninstitutionalized elderly are marginally deficient as compared to younger subjects. The data does not sufficiently characterize the subjects as to alcoholism.

Thiamin status can also be evaluated in terms of the functional adequacy of TPP-dependent enzymes. Transketolase data show clearly that some impairment is present in geriatric patients particularly with concomitant disease. Thus, *Brin* et al. [31] found 7% severely depleted in a Veterans Administration Hospital population and, in another study [32], found 50% depleted in a nursing home. *Hoorn* et al. [67] found 23% depleted in the Netherlands while *Vir and Love* [135] found 13 to 18% in Ireland.

The possibility that some elderly patients are functionally thiamin-deficient because of an intrinsic abnormality of one or another thiamin-dependent enzyme is of great interest. Individuals who maintain a persistent abnormality of an enzymatic index of thiamin nutrition despite adequate repletion with the vitamin should be intensively studied biochemically.

The clinical importance of thiamin as a cause of illness in older North Americans and Europeans is uncertain, but has a substantial likelihood of being important only in alcoholics. In the tropics it is more likely that the elderly population is more depleted, for thiamin supplementation is less available and the indigenous intestinal changes interfere with its availability.

In all parts of the world it is difficult to assess where illness begins and 'age-dependent loss of function' ends. Heart failure, neuropathy, and loss of higher intellectual function are all common in the elderly and may or may not be accelerated by concomitant diminution in thiamin availability.

XI. Thiamin Toxicity

Thiamin is generally regarded as safe and nontoxic in any amount. Doses in excess of 50 mg/kg or in an adult in excess of 3 g daily may be toxic. Thiamin overdosage has been reported [99]. A 47-year-old woman ingesting 10 g of thiamin daily for 2.5 weeks developed headache, irritability, insomnia, tachycardia and generalized weakness. Symptoms disappeared within 2 days of discontinuing thiamin. 1 week later, the patient resumed thiamin at a dose of 5 g daily and after 4.5 weeks symptoms recurred.

In rodents, the LD_{50} for thiamin varies from 75 to 200 mg/kg i.v. to approximately 3,000 mg/kg orally. The size of the oral dose in part is due to an absorption barrier. Shock, muscle tremor, convulsion and respiratory disturbances precede death. Thiamin up to 50 mg/kg/day did not affect either fertility, size of litters, or rate of fetal malformation in rodents [119].

Hypersensitivity to thiamin has been found. *Combes and Groopman* [42] reported 2 cases of contact dermatitis in female pharmaceutical workers (aged 35 and 36) who worked filling ampules of thiamin. Dermatitis appeared 3 and 8 months after initial exposure. A patchy erythematovesicular dermatitis covering fingers, hands, wrists, and forearms was present with the unusual feature of fine scales over the involved areas. Both women had positive patch tests.

A generalized eczema was observed in a 17-year-old woman working in a pharmaceutical firm with multiple agents. A patch test was positive for thiamin and the process disappeared when she changed employment. A relapse occurred after ingestion of 200 mg of thiamin and intracutaneous injection of 10 mg of the vitamin [65].

A possible hypersensitivity death occurred in a 55-year-old women who took 100 mg thiamin HCl daily for 15 days with no reaction. 2 months later she took one 100-mg tablet and within 1 day was hospitalized with acute skin rash and pruritis over her entire body. Chest pain, dyspnea, and choking sensations were prominent. Despite treatment with noradrenaline, hydrocortisone and epinephrine, the patient died the next day. Autopsy revealed only pulmonary edema and the skin lesions [2].

Oral administration of thiamin was thought to account for the development of encephalitis in a 25-year-old man. A severe skin rash accompanied this reaction [91].

XII. Conclusions

(1) The dietary intake of free-living elderly Americans seems adequate with regard to thiamin. About 25% of Americans in older age groups do not achieve RDA intake due in large measure to reduced calorie intake. Thiamin intake for each 1,000 kcal seems adequate for nearly all free-living non-alcoholic Americans. In all other parts of the world this is not true because cereals are not supplemented.

(2) Severe disease increasingly interferes with the dietary intake of thiamin.

(3) Thiamin status judged by blood thiamin or transketolase levels in erythrocytes of free-living healthy North Americans seems to be normal. No widespread clinical syndromes clearly attributable to thiamin deficiency are described. Up to 10% of selected elderly populations do have deficient thiamin nutrition by biochemical criteria – usually these are in poor or ill populations. This figure will be higher in all parts of the world.

(4) Alcoholism interferes with absorption of thiamin in a major way. This absorptive defect in alcoholism is coupled with a diminished dietary

intake and an increased metabolic demand which cause alcoholism to be in all age groups overwhelmingly the most significant precipitant of clinically meaningful thiamin deficiency in a North American population.

(5) Folate deficiency, common in the tropics, would be expected to be as important as alcoholism.

(6) No clinical syndrome or constellation of findings is sufficiently common in the elderly with thiamin deficiency to strongly suggest this diagnosis. The changes of aging and the known changes of thiamin deficiency are similar and are not distinctive. The incidence of thiamin responsive lesions in aging nonalcoholic populations is invariably less than 1%.

XIII. Areas of High Priority Investigation

(1) Studies of thiamin requirements on aging animal populations are needed. Emphasis should be placed on CNS and cardiac function with regard to thiamin status and the function of thiamin-dependent enzyme systems.

(2) More data is needed on alcohol consumption and its relation to thiamin status in older populations in representative areas of the world.

(3) Better methods are needed for surveying multiple TPP and thiamin triphosphate enzyme systems in man.

(4) Clarification is needed of the role of thiamin triphosphate in CNS function and its importance in the membrane function. Clarification of presence or absence of inhibitors of this function and their significance is also needed.

(5) Careful assessment of altered enzyme binding of thiamin in elderly patients with depletion states and the genetic basis of such alterations if present is needed. Extensive assays of the multiple thiamin-dependent enzyme systems to determine the prevalence of heterozygotic forms of those genetically determined enzyme variants for which severe neurological disease has been described in the homozygous forms. The clinical relevance of these heterozygous states must be evaluated. Detailed studies of the biochemical binding properties of thiamin-dependent enzymes in those rare humans who fail to replete with oral replacement would also be helpful.

(6) Broad prospective neurological and psychological surveys are needed to determine which symptoms and signs in elderly thiamin-deficient patients are responsive to thiamin replacement and to determine the natural history of that responsiveness. Elderly dizziness, aberration

of vibratory sense, change in nerve conduction time, muscle cramps, memory loss, and psychiatric parameters are among those which need to be evaluated.

(7) Development of better biochemical methods to determine thiamin levels in blood and urine and to evaluate status of thiamin-dependent enzyme systems is essential.

References

1 Abraham, S.; Carroll, M.D.; Dresser, C.M.; Johnson, C.L.: National Center for Health Statistics: caloric and selected nutrient values for persons 1–74 years of age, United States 1971–1974, Vital and Health Statistics Series 11–No. 209 DHEW publ. No. (DHS) 79–1657 (US Government Printing Office, Washington 1979).

2 Acharya, V.; Store, S.D.; Golwalla, A.F.: Anaphylaxis following ingestion of aneurine hydrochloride. J. Indian med. Ass. *52:* 84–85 (1969).

3 Adams, R.D.; Victor, M.: Principles of neurology; 2nd ed. (McGraw-Hill, New York 1981).

4 Airth, R.L.; Foerster, G.E.: Simultaneous determination of thiamine and pyrithiamine. Methods Enzymol. *18a:* 81–86 (1970).

5 Akbarian, M.; Dreyfus, P.M.: Blood transketolase activity in beriberi heart disease. J. Am. med. Ass. *203:* 77–80 (1968).

6 Akbarian, M.; Yankopoulos, N.A.; Abelmann, W.H.: Hemodynamic studies in beriberi heart disease. Am. J. Med. *41:* 197–212 (1966).

7 Alexander, B.; Landwehr, G.: Studies of thiamine metabolism in man. I.Thiamine balance. The normal requirement of vitamin B_1 and the role of fecal thiamine in human nutrition. J. clin. Invest. *25:* 287–293 (1946).

8 Alexander, C.S.: Nutritional heart disease. Cardiovasc. Clin. *4:* 221 (1972).

9 Almy, T.P.: Factors leading to digestive disorders in the elderly. Bull. N.Y. Acad. Med. *57:* 709–717 (1981).

10 Ariaey-Nejad, M.R.; Balaghi, M.; Baker, E.M.; Sauberlich, H.E.: Thiamin metabolism in man. Am. J. clin. Nutr. *23:* 764–778 (1970).

11 Atlas, M.; Hanley, H.G.; Stultz, D.; Jones, M.R.; McAllister, R.G.: Fulminant beriberi heart disease with lactic acidosis: presentation of a case with evaluation of left ventricular function and review of pathophysiologic mechanisms. Circulation *58:* 566–572 (1978).

12 Baczyk, S.; Szwajca, T.: Determination of thiamine in biological material. Mikrochim. Acta *2:* 545–549 (1977).

13 Baker, E.M.; Balaghi, M.; Pardini, R.S.; Sauberlich, H.E.: Metabolism of 2-^{14}C-thiazole labeled thiamine in man. Fed. Proc. *25:* 245 (1966).

14 Baker, H.: Discussion. Am. J. clin. Nutr. *20:* 543–546 (1967).

15 Baker, H.; Frank, O.; Hutner, S.H.: Vitamin analyses in medicine; in Goodhart, Shils, Modern nutrition in health and disease; 6th ed., pp. 611–640 (Lea & Febiger, New York 1980).

16 Baker, H.; Frank, O.; Thind, I.S.; Jaslow, S.P.; Louria, D.B.: Vitamin profiles in

elderly persons living at home or in nursing homes, versus profile in healthy young subjects. J. Am. Geriat. Soc. *27:* 444–450 (1979).

17 Baker, H.; Frank, O.; Jaslow, S.P.: Oral versus intramuscular vitamin supplementation for hypovitaminosis in the elderly. J. Am. Geriat. Soc. *28:* 42–45 (1980).

18 Balaghi, M.; Pearson, W.N.: Intracellular distribution of radioactive thiamine in normal and thiamine deficient rats. Fed. Proc. *25:* 245 (1966).

19 Balaghi, M.; Pearson, W.N.: Metabolism of physiological doses of thiazole-2-^{14}C-labeled thiamine by the rat. J. Nutr. *89:* 265–270 (1966).

20 Bamji, M.S.: Transketolase activity and urinary excretion of thiamin in the assessment of thiamin-nutrition status of Indians. Am. J. clin. Nutr. *23:* 52–58 (1970).

21 Barchi, R.L.: The non-metabolic role of thiamin in excitable membrane function; in Gubler, Fijiwara, Dreyfus, Thiamine (Wiley, New York 1976).

22 Berman, K.; Fishman, R.A.: Thiamine phosphate metabolism and possible coenzyme-independent functions of thiamine in brain. J. Neurochem. *24:* 457–465 (1975).

23 Birchfield, R.I.: Postural hypotension in Wernicke's disease: a manifestation of autonomic nervous system involvement. Am. J. Med. *36:* 404–414 (1964).

24 Blass, J.P.: Disorders of pyruvate metabolism. Neurology, N.Y. *29:* 280–286 (1979).

25 Blass, J.P.; Avigan, J.; Uhlendorf, B.W.: A defect in pyruvate decarboxylase in a child with an intermittent movement disorder. J. clin. Invest. *49:* 423–432 (1970).

26 Blass, J.P.; Cederbaum, S.D.; Kark, R.A.P.: Rapid diagnosis of pyruvate and ketoglutarate dehydrogenase deficiencies in platelet-enriched preparations from blood. Clinica chim. Acta *75:* 21–30 (1977).

27 Blass, J.P.; Gibson, G.E.: Genetic factors in Wernicke-Korsakoff syndrome. Alcoholism *3:* 126–134 (1979).

28 Blass, J.P.; Gibson, G.E.: Abnormality of a thiamine-requiring enzyme in patients with Wernicke-Korsakoff syndrome. New Engl. J. Med. *297:* 1367–1370 (1977).

29 Braunwald, E.: Heart disease, a textbook of cardiovascular medicine (Saunders, Philadelphia 1980).

30 Brin, M.: Erythrocyte transketolase in early thiamine deficiency. Ann. N.Y. Acad. Sci. *98:* 528–541 (1962).

31 Brin, M.; Dibble, M.V.; Peel, A.; McMullen, E.; Bourquin, A.; Chen, N.: Some preliminary findings on the nutritional status of the aged in Onondaga County, New York. Am. J. clin. Nutr. *17:* 7240–7258 (1965).

32 Brin, M.; Schwartzberg, S.H.; Arthur-Davis, D.: A vitamin evaluation program as applied to 10 elderly residents in a community home for the aged. J. Am. Geriat. Soc. *12:* 493–499 (1964).

33 Brin, M.; Shohet, S.S.; Davidson, C.S.: Effect of thiamin deficiency on mammalian erythrocyte metabolism. Fed. Proc. *15:* 224 (1956).

34 Brin, M.; Shohet, S.S.; Davidson, C.S.: The effect of thiamine deficiency on the glucose oxidative pathway of rat erythrocytes. J. biol. Chem. *230:* 319–326 (1958).

35 Brubacher, G.; Haenel, A.; Ritzel, G.: Transketolase activity, thiamine excretion, and blood thiamine content in man as criteria of vitamin B_1 supply. Int. J. Vitam. Nutr. Res. *42:* 190–195 (1972).

36 Burwell, C.S.; Dexter, L.: Beri-beri heart disease. Trans. Ass. Am. Physns *60:* 59–64 (1947).

37 Butters, N.; Cermak, L.S.: Alcoholic Korsakoff's syndrome. An information-processing approach to amnesia (Academic Press, New York 1980).
38 Campbell, J.A.; Morrison, A.B.: Some factors affecting the absorption of vitamins. Am. J. clin. Nutr. *12:* 162–169 (1963).
39 Carroll, M.D.; Abraham, S.; Dresser, C.M.: National Center for Health Statistics: dietary intake source data, United States 1976–1980, Vital and Health Statistics Series II (Public Health Service, DHHS, US Government Printing Office, Hyattsville 1982).
40 Cline, J.K.; Williams, R.R.; Finkelstein, J.: Studies of crystalline vitamin B_1. XVII. Synthesis of vitamin B_1. J. Am. Chem. Soc. *59:* 1052–1054 (1937).
41 Cole, M.; Turner, A.; Frank, O.; Baker, H.; Leevy, C.M.: Extraocular palsy and thiamine therapy in Wernicke's encephalopathy. Am. J. clin. Nutr. *22:* 44–51 (1969).
42 Combes, F.C.; Groopman, J.: Contact dermatitis due to thiamine. Report of two cases. Archs Derm. Syph. *61:* 858–859 (1950).
43 Cooper, J.R.; Pincus, J.H.: Substrate necrotizing encephalomyelitis; in Gubler, Fujiwara, Dreyfus, Thiamine (Wiley, New York 1976).
44 Cooper, J.R.; Pincus, J.H.: The role of thiamine in nervous tissue. Neurochem. Res. *4:* 223–239 (1979).
45 Dancis, J.; Hutzler, J.; Levitz, M.: The diagnosis of maple syrup urine disease (branched-chain ketoaciduria) by the in vitro study of the peripheral leukocyte. Pediatrics, Springfield *32:* 234–238 (1963).
46 Danner, D.J.; Lemmon, S.K.; Elsas, L.J., II: Stabilization of mammalian liver branched-chain alpha-ketoacid dehydrogenase by thiamin pyrophosphate. Archs Biochem. Biophys. *202:* 23–28 (1980).
47 Danner, D.J.; Wheeler, F.B.; Lemmon, S.K.; Elsas, L.J., II: In vivo and in vitro response of human branched chain, alpha-ketoacid dehydrogenase to thiamine and thiamine pyrophosphate. Pediat. Res. *12:* 235–238 (1978).
48 Dunn, T.B.; Morris, H.P.; Dubnik, C.S.: Lesions of chronic thiamine deficiency in mice. J. natn. Cancer Inst. *8:* 139–155 (1947).
49 Elsas, L.J., II; Danner, D.J.: The role of thiamin in maple syrup urine disease. Ann. N.Y. Acad. Sci. *378:* 404–421 (1982).
50 Elsom, K.O.; Reinhold, J.G.; Nicholson, J.T.L.; Chornock, C.: Studies of the B vitamins in the human subject. V. The normal requirement for thiamine; some factors influencing its utilization and excretion. Am. J. med. Sci. *203:* 569–577 (1942).
51 Engel, R.W.; Phillips, P.H.: The lack of nerve degeneration in uncomplicated vitamin B_1 deficiency in the chick and the rat. J. Nutr. *16:* 585–596 (1938).
52 Fennelly, J.; Frank, O.; Baker, H.; Leevy, C.M.: Red blood cell transketolase activity in malnourished alcoholics with cirrhosis. Am. J. clin. Nutr. *20:* 946–949 (1967).
53 Fisher, M.: Residual neuropathological changes in Canadians held prisoners of war by the Japanese. Can. Serv. med. J. *11:* 157–199 (1955).
54 Follis, R.H.: Deficiency disease (Thomas, Springfield 1958).
55 Friedmann, T.E.; Kmieciak, T.C.; Keegan, P.K.; Sheet, B.B.: The absorption, destruction, and excretion of orally administered thiamin by human subjects. Gastroenterology *11:* 100–114 (1948).
56 Ghez, C.: Vestibular paresis: a clinical feature of Wernicke's disease. J. Neurol. Neurosurg. Psychiat. *32:* 134–139 (1969).

57 Gibson, G.; Barclay, L.; Blass, J.: The role of the cholinergic system in thiamin deficiency. Ann. N.Y. Acad. Sci. *378:* 383–403 (1982).

58 Grandjean, A.C.; Korth, L.L.; Kara, G.C.; Smith, J.L.; Schaefer, A.E.: Nutritional status of elderly participants in a congregate meals programs. J. Am. diet. Ass. *78:* 324–329 (1981).

59 Griffiths, L.L.; Brocklehurst, J.C.; Scott, D.L.; Marks, J.; Blackley, J.: Thiamine and ascorbic acid levels in the elderly. Geront. clin. *9:* 1–10 (1967).

60 Harrill, I.; Cervone, N.: Vitamin status of older women. Am. J. clin. Nutr. *30:* 431–440 (1977).

61 Harris, R.S.; Jansen, B.C.P.; Wuest, H.M.; et al.: in Sebrell, Harris, Thiamine, pp. 97–164 (Academic Press, New York 1972).

62 Hell, D.; Six, P.; Salkeld, R.: Vitamin B_1 deficiency in chronic alcoholics and its clinical correlation. Schweiz. med. Wschr. *106:* 1466–1470 (1976).

63 Hennessy, D.J.; Cerecedo, L.R.: The determination of free and phosphorylated thiamin by a modified thiochrome assay. J. Am. Chem. Soc. *61:* 179–183 (1939).

64 Hilker, D.M.; Chan, K.C.; Chen, R.; Smith, R.L.: Anti-thiamin effects of tea. Temperature and pH dependence. Nutr. Rep. int. *4:* 223 (1971).

65 Hjorth, N.: Contact dermatitis from vitamin B_1 (thiamine): relapse after ingestion of thiamine. Cross-sensitization to co-carboxylase. J. invest. Derm. *30:* 261–264 (1958).

66 Hohn, P.; Gabbert, H.; Wagner, R.D.: Differentiation and aging of the rat intestinal mucosa. II. Morphological enzyme histochemical and dise electrophoretic aspects of the aging of the small intestinal mucosa. Diet Aging Devel. *7:* 217–222 (1979).

67 Hoorn, R.K.J.; Filkweert, J.P.; Westerink, D.: Vitamin B_1, B_2 and B_6 deficiencies in geriatric patients, measured by coenzyme stimulation of enzyme activities. Clinica chim. Acta *61:* 151–162 (1975).

68 Horecker, B.L.; Smyrniotis, P.Z.: The coenzyme function of thiamine pyrophosphate in pentose phosphate metabolism. J. Am. Chem. Soc. *75:* 1009–1010 (1953).

69 Hoyumpa, A.M., Jr.; Breen, K.J.; Schenker, S.; Wilson, F.A.: Thiamine transport across the rat intestine. II. Effect of ethanol. J. Lab. clin. Med. *86:* 803–816 (1975).

70 Hoyumpa, A.M., Jr.; Middleton, H.M., III; Wilson, F.A.; Schenker, S.: Thiamine transport across the rat intestine. I. Normal characteristics. Gastroenterology *68:* 1218–1227 (1975).

71 Hurst, J.W.: The heart; 4th ed. (McGraw-Hill, New York 1978).

72 Iber, F.L.; Blass, J.P.; Brin, M.; Leevy, C.M.: Thiamin in the elderly – relation to alcoholism and to neurological degenerative disease. Am. J. clin. Nutr. *36:* 1067–1082 (1982).

73 Ikram, H.; Maslowski, A.H.; Smith, B.L.; Nicholls, M.G.: The haemodynamic, histopathological and hormonal features of alcoholic cardiac beriberi. Q. Jl Med. *200:* 359–375 (1981).

74 Interdepartmental Committee on Nutrition for National Defense. Nutrition Survey Union of Burma (US Government Printing Office, Washington 1963).

75 Itokawa, Y.; Schulz, A.R.; Cooper, J.R.: Thiamine in nerve membranes. Biochim. biophys. Acta *266:* 293 (1972).

76 Jordan, F.; Chen, G.; Nishikawa, S.; Wu, B.S.: Potential roles of the aminopyrimidine ring in thiamine catalyzed reactions. Ann. N.Y. Acad. Sci. *378:* 14–31 (1982).

77 Justice, C.L.; Howe, J.M.; Clark, H.E.: Study in a private nursing home. Dietary intakes and nutritional status of elderly patients. J. Am. diet. Ass. *65:* 639–646 (1974).

78 Kawai, C.; Wakabayashi, A.; Matsumura, T.; Yui, Y.: Reappearance of beriberi heart disease in Japan. A study of 23 cases. Am. J. Med. *69:* 383–386 (1980).

79 Klatsky, A.L.; Friedman, G.D.; Siegelaub, A.B.; Gerard, M.J.: Alcohol consumption among white, black, or oriental men and women: Kaiser-Permanente multiphasic health examination data. Am. J. Epidem. *105:* 311–323 (1977).

80 Klipstein, F.: Tropical sprue; in Bochus, Gastroenterology, vol. 2, pp. 285–305 (Saunders, Philadelphia 1976).

81 Ksiezak-Reding, H.; Blass, J.P.; Gibson, G.E.: Studies on the pyruvate dehydrogenase complex in brain with the arylamine acetyltransferase coupled assay. J. Neurochem. (in press).

82 Leevy, C.M.: Thiamine deficiency and alcoholism. Ann. N.Y. Acad. Sci. *378:* 316–326 (1982).

83 Leevy, C.M.; Baker, H.; TenHove, W.; Frank, O.; Cherrick, G.R.: B-complex vitamins in liver disease of the alcoholic. Am. J. clin. Nutr. *16:* 339–346 (1965).

84 Leevy, C.M.; Cardi, L.; Frank, O.; Gellene, R.; Baker, H.: Incidence and significance of hypovitaminemia in a randomly selected municipal hospital population. Am. J. clin. Nutr. *17:* 259–271 (1965).

85 Leichter, J.; Angel, J.F.; Lee, M.: Nutritional status of a select group of free-living elderly people in Vancouver. Can. med. Ass. J. *118:* 40–43 (1978).

86 Lindenbaum, J.: Tropical enteropathy. Gastroenterology *64:* 637–652 (1973).

87 Lindenbaum, J.; Gerson, C.D.; Kent, T.H.: Recovery of small-intestinal structure and function after residence in the tropics. I. Studies in Peace Corps Volunteers. Ann. intern. Med. *74:* 218–222 (1971).

88 Lindenbaum, J.; Kent, T.H.; Sprinz, H.: Malabsorption and jejunitis in American Peace Corps Volunteers in Pakistan. Ann. intern. Med. *65:* 1201–1209 (1966).

89 Lyons, J.S.; Trulson, M.F.: Food practices of older people living at home. J. Geront. *11:* 66–72 (1956).

90 Mair, R.; Capra, C.; McEntree, W.J.; Engen, T.: Odor discrimination and memory in Korsakoff's psychosis. J. exp. Psychol. *6:* 445–458 (1980).

91 Markiewicz, M.; Uss, B.Z.: Encephalitis as a consequence of allergy to vitamin B_1. Polski Tyg. Lek. *25:* 1661–1662 (1970).

92 Markkanen, T.; Heilkinheimo, R.; Dahl, M.: Transketolase activity of red blood cells from infancy to old age. Acta haemat. *42:* 148–153 (1969).

93 May, J.M.; McLellan, D.L. (eds): Ecology of malnutrition in Middle Africa: Ghana, Nigeria, Republic of the Congo, Rwanda and Burundi and the former French Equatorial Africa (Hafner, New York 1965).

94 May, J.M.; McLellan, D.L. (eds): Ecology of malnutrition in Eastern Africa: Equitorial Guinea, the Gambia, Liberia, Sierra Leone, Malawi, Rhodesia, Zambia, Kenya, Tanzania, Uganda, Ethiopia, the French territory of the Atars and Issas, the Somali Republic and Sudan (Hafner, New York 1970).

95 May, J.M.; McLellan, D.L. (eds): Ecology of malnutrition in Seven Countries of Southern Africa and in Portuguese Guinea: The Republic of Southern Africa, South West Africa (Namibia), Botswana, Lesotho, Swaziland, Mozambique, Angola, Portuguese Guinea (Hafner, New York 1971).

96 Melnick, D.; Hochberg, M.; Oser, B.L.: Physiological availability of the vitamins. I. The human bioassay technic. J. Nutr. *30:* 67–79 (1945).
97 Meshi, T.; Sato, Y.: Hydrolytic cleavage of thiamine in mammalian animals. Chem. pharm. Bull., Tokyo *14:* 1444–1448 (1966).
98 Mezey, E.: Intestinal function in chronic alcoholism. Ann. N.Y. Acad. Sci. *252:* 215–227 (1975).
99 Mills, C.A.: Thiamine overdosage and toxicity. J. Am. med. Ass. *116:* 2101 (1941).
100 Morson, B.C.; Dawson, I.M.P.: Gastrointestinal pathology, 2nd ed. (Blackwell, Oxford 1979).
101 Najjar, V.A.; Holt, L.E., Jr.: The biosynthesis of thiamine in man and its implications in human nutrition. J. Am. med. Ass. *123:* 683–684 (1943).
102 Neal, R.A.; Pearson, W.N.: Studies of thiamine metabolism in the rat. I. Metabolic products found in urine. J. Nutr. *83:* 343–350 (1964).
103 Nutrition Survey in the Kingdom of Thailand. A report by ICNND, 1962, pp. 32–36.
104 Nutrition Survey in the Republic of Vietnam. A report by ICNND, 1960, p. 3.
105 Nutrition Survey in the Federation of Malaya. A report by ICNND, 1964, pp. 61, 129.
106 Oldham, H.G.; Davis, M.V.; Roberts, L.J.: Thiamine excretions and blood levels of young women on diets containing varying levels of the B vitamins, with some observations on niacin and pantothenic acid. J. Nutr. *32:* 163–179 (1944).
107 Pearson, W.N.: Thiamin; in Gyorgy, Pearson, The vitamins; 2nd ed., vol. VII, pp. 53–98 (Academic Press, New York 1967).
108 Pincus, J.H.; Cooper, J.R.; Piros, K.; Turner, V.: Specificity of the urine inhibitor test for Leigh's disease. Neurology, Minneap. *24:* 885–890 (1974).
109 Plaitakis, A.; Hwang, E.C.; Van Woert, M.H.; Szilagyi, P.I.A.; Berl, S.: Effect of thiamin deficiency on brain neurotransmitter systems. Ann. N.Y. Acad. Sci. *378:* 367–381 (1982).
110 Racker, E.; DeLaHaba, G.; Leder, I.G.: Thiamine pyrophosphate, a coenzyme of transketolase. J. Am. Chem. Soc. *75:* 1010–1011 (1953).
111 Rindi, G.; DeGiuseppe, L.: A new chromatographic method for the determination of thiamine and its mono-, di- and tri-phosphates in animal tissues. Biochem. J. *78:* 602–606 (1961).
112 Rindi, G.; Ventura, U.: Thiamin intestinal transport. Physiol. Rev. *52:* 821–827 (1972).
113 Rinehart, J.F.; Friedman, M.; Greenberg, L.D.: Effect of experimental thiamin deficiency on the nervous system of the Rhesus monkey. Archs Path. *48:* 129–139 (1949).
114 Roine, P.; Koivula, L.; Pekkarinen, M.: Plasma vitamin C level and erythrocyte transketolase activity compared with vitamin intakes among old people in Finland. Nutrition *4:* 116–120 (1972).
115 Rowlands, D.T., Jr.; Vilter, C.F.: A study of the cardiac stigmata in prolonged human thiamine deficiency. Circulation *21:* 4–12 (1960).
116 Ruenwongsa, P.; Cooper, J.R.: The role of bound thiamine pyrophosphate in the synthesis of thiamine triphosphate in rat liver. Biochim. biophys. Acta *482:* 64–70 (1977).
117 Sauberlich, H.E.; Herman, Y.F.; Stevens, C.O.; Herman, R.H.: Thiamin requirement of the adult human. Am. J. clin. Nutr. *32:* 2237–2248 (1979).

118 Schuckit, M.A.; Pastor, P.A., Jr.: The elderly as a unique population: alcoholism. Alcoholism *2:* 31–38 (1978).

119 Scientific literature reviews on generally recognized as safe (GRAS) food ingredients – thiamine (US Food and Drug Administration, Washington 1974).

120 Somogyi, J.C.; Nageli, U.: Antithiamine effect of coffee. Int. J. Vitam. Nutr. Res. *46:* 149–153 (1976).

121 Stefadouros, M.A.; El Shahawy, M.; Witham, A.C.: Shoshin in Georgia; a case of acute fulminant cardiac beriberi. J. Med. Ass. Ga. *65:* 149–152 (1976).

122 Stiedemann, M.; Jansen, C.; Harrill, I.: Nutritional status of elderly men and women. J. Am. diet. Ass. *73:* 132–139 (1978).

123 Strauss, M.B.: The etiology of 'alcoholic' polyneuritis. Am. J. med. Sci. *189:* 378–382 (1935).

124 Thomson, A.D.; Baker, H.; Leevy, C.M.: Patterns of ^{35}S-thiamine hydrochloride absorption in the malnourished alcoholic patient. J. Lab. clin. Med. *76:* 34–45 (1970).

125 Thomson, A.D.; Baker, H.; Leevy, C.M.: Thiamine absorption in alcoholism. Am. J. clin. Nutr. *21:* 537–538 (1968).

126 Thomson, A.D.; Frank, O.; Baker, H.; Leevy, C.M.: Thiamine propyl disulfide: absorption and utilization. Ann. intern. Med. *74:* 529–534 (1971).

127 Thomson, A.D.; Leevy, C.M.: Observations on the mechanism of thiamine hydrochloride absorption in man. Clin. Sci. *43:* 153–163 (1972).

128 Tomasulo, P.A.; Kater, R.M.H.; Iber, F.L.: Impairment of thiamine absorption in alcoholism. Am. J. clin. Nutr. *21:* 1341–1344 (1968).

129 Verrett, M.J.; Cerecedo, L.R.: Metabolism of thiamine-S^{35} in the rabbit. Proc. Soc. exp. Biol. Med. *98:* 509–513 (1958).

130 Victor, M.; Adams, R.D.: On the etiology of the alcoholic neurologic diseases: with special reference to the role of nutrition. Am. J. clin. Nutr. *9:* 379–397 (1961).

131 Victor, M.; Adams, R.D.; Collins, G.H.: The Wernicke-Korsakoff syndrome, a clinical and pathological study of 245 patients, 82 with post-mortem examinations, pp. 2–13 (Davis, Philadelphia 1971).

132 Vimokesant, S.: Beriberi caused by antithiamin factors in food and its prevention. Ann. N.Y. Acad. Sci. *378:* 123–126 (1982).

133 Vimokesant, S.L.; Hilker, D.M.; Nakornchai, S.; Rungruangsak, K.; Dhanamitta, S.: Effect of betel nut and fermented fish on the thiamin status of northeastern Thais. Am. J. clin. Nutr. *28:* 1458–1463 (1975).

134 Vimokesant, S.L.; Nakornchai, S.; Dhanamita, S.; Hiken, D.M.: Effect of tea consumption on thiamin status in man. Nutr. Rep. int. *9:* 372–375 (1974).

135 Vir, S.C.; Love, A.H.G.: Nutritional status of institutionalized and non-institutionalized aged in Belfast, Northern Ireland. Am. J. clin. Nutr. *32:* 1934–1947 (1979).

136 Wada, T.; Takagi, H.; Minakami, H.; et al.: A new thiamin derivative, *S*-benzoylthiamine *O*-monophosphate. Science *134:* 195–196 (1961).

137 Wagner, P.I.: Beriberi heart disease. Physiologic data and difficulties in diagnosis. Am. Heart J. *69:* 200–205 (1965).

138 Warburg, O.; Christian, W.: Über das gelbe Ferment und seine Wirkungen. Biochem. Z. *266:* 377–411 (1933).

139 Warren, P.M.; Pepperman, M.A.; Montgomery, R.D.: Age changes in small intestinal mucosa. Lancet *ii:* 849–850 (1978).

140 Weiss, S.: Occidental beriberi with cardiovascular manifestations. Its relation to thiamin deficiency. J. Am. med. Ass. *115:* 832–839 (1940).

141 Wick, H.; Schweizer, K.; Baumgartner, R.: Thiamine dependency in a patient with congenital lacticacidaemia due to pyruvate dehydrogenase deficiency. Agents Actions *7:* 405–410 (1977).

142 Williams, R.D.; Mason, H.L.; Power, M.H.; Wilder, R.M.: Induced thiamine (vitamin B_1) deficiency in man: relation of depletion of thiamine to development of biochemical defect and or polyneuropathy. Archs intern. Med. *71:* 38–53 (1943).

143 Williams, R.D.; Mason, H.L.; Smith, B.F.; Wilder, R.M.: Induced thiamine (vitamin B_1) deficiency and the thiamine requirement of man. Archs intern. Med. *69:* 721–738 (1942).

144 Williams, R.D.; Mason, H.L.; Wilder, R.M.; Smith, B.F.: Observations on induced thiamine (vitamin B_1) deficiency in man. Archs intern. Med. *66:* 785–799 (1940).

145 Williams, R.H.; Bissell, G.W.; Peters, J.B.: Thiamine metabolism with particular reference to the role of the liver and kidneys. Archs intern. Med. *73:* 203–211 (1944).

146 Williams, R.R.: Structure of vitamin B. J. Am. chem. Soc. *57:* 229–230 (1935).

147 Yearick, E.S.; Wang, M.L.; Pisias, S.J.: Nutritional status of the elderly: dietary and biochemical findings. J. Geront. *35:* 663–671 (1980).

148 Yusa, T.; Maruo, B.: Biochemical role of thiamine triphosphoric acid ester. J. Biochem. *60:* 735–737 (1966).

149 Zimberg, S.: The elderly alcoholic. Gerontologist *14:* 221–224 (1974).

150 Ziporin, Z.Z.; Nunes, W.T.; Powell, R.C.; Waring, P.P.; Sauberlich, H.E.: Excretion of thiamine and its metabolites in the urine of young adult males receiving restricted intakes of the vitamin. J. Nutr. *85:* 287–296 (1965).

F.L. Iber, MD, Chief, Division of Gastroenterology,
Veterans Administration Medical Center,
3900 Loch Raven Boulevard, Baltimore, MD 21218 (USA)

Wld Rev. Nutr. Diet., vol. 44, pp. 117–154 (Karger, Basel 1984)

Cholesterol Autoxidation, Health and Arteriosclerosis

A Review on Situations in Developed Countries[1]

Shi-Kaung Peng, C. Bruce Taylor

Department of Pathology, Harbor-UCLA Medical Center, Torrance, Calif., and Research Service, V.A. Medical Center, Albany, N.Y., USA

Contents

Introduction

Although 9 years before, *Anitschkow* [1] in 1913, first described the production of the typical picture of atherosclerosis in rabbits by feeding what he presumed to be pure cholesterol dissolved in vegetable oil, *Schulze and Winterstein* [2] in 1904 had already noted that crystalline cholesterol could undergo autoxidation in the presence of air, but the reaction products

[1] This work was supported by the Medical Research Service of the Veterans Administration, and the American Heart Association, Northeastern New York Chapter, Grant No. 210031.

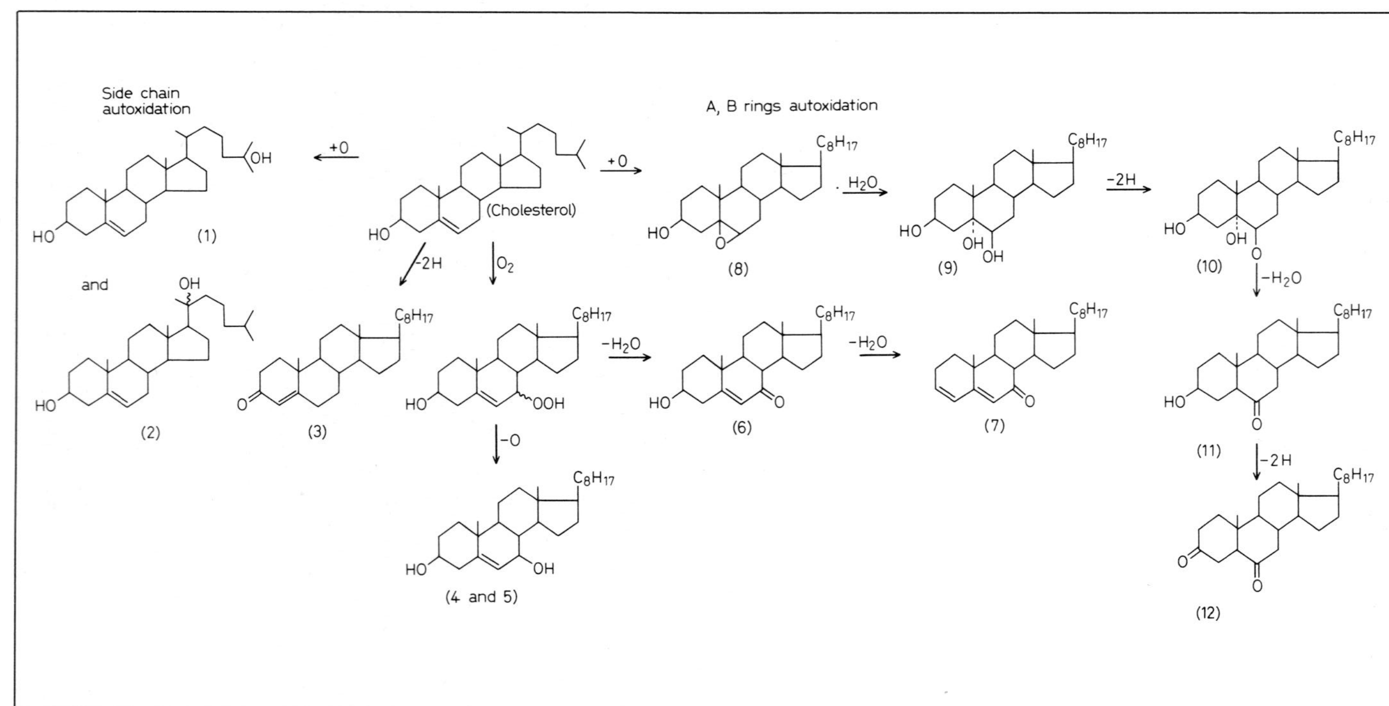

Fig. 1. Mechanisms and products of cholesterol autoxidation: (1) 25-hydroxycholesterol; (2) 20α-hydroxycholesterol; (3) 4-cholesten-3-one; (4) 7α-hydroxycholesterol; (5) 7β-hydroxycholesterol; (6) 7-ketocholesterol; (7) 3,5-cholestedien-7-one; (8) 5,6-epoxycholesterol; (9) cholestane-3β,5α,6β-triol; (10) cholestan-3β,5α-diol-6-one; (11) cholestan-3β,ol-6-one; (12) cholestan-3,6-dione.

were not identified. Since then many other investigators have found that the occurrence of spontaneous oxidation of cholesterol is related to heat [3–6], light and radiation [7–9]. *Lifschutz,* reviewed by *Bergstrom and Samuelsson* [10], was the first investigator who observed the presence of 'oxycholesterol' when a solution of cholesterol in acetic acid was treated with a little benzoyl peroxide and heated briefly; a product in this solution gave an intensive blue or green color on addition of sulfuric acid. Later *Lifschutz* reported the discovery of preformed 'oxycholesterol' in the nonsaponified fractions of blood and tissues.

The mechanisms of autoxidation have been extensively studied [10–14]. The types of oxidation products appear to be dependent upon the physical state of cholesterol. When cholesterol is in a dispersed state or in an aqueous colloidal solution, the A, B rings, particularly the 5,6-double bond, seem to be the most reactive positions and yield oxidation products such as α and β isomers of 7-hydroxycholesterol, 7-ketocholesterol, cholesta-3,4-diene-7-one via free radical reactions and formation of 7–hydroperoxide involving initial allylic C-7 hydrogen abstraction and reaction with ground state dioxygen ($^3O_2$) to yield C-7 peroxyl radicals [12, 13] and cholestane-3β,5α,6β-triol, cholestane-3β,5α-diol-6-one, cholestane-3,6-dione via 5,6-epoxide [14]. On the other hand, when cholesterol is in the crystalline state and in the presence of air, the oxidation reaction is governed by the arrangement of molecules in the crystal, i.e. in the double layer with the 3-hydroxyl group in juxtaposition and the side chain exposed. The molecules are evidently closely packed to prevent the attack of oxygen at the A, B rings and the attack is instead towards the tertiary 20 and 25 carbon positions. *Fieser* et al. [15] studied the impurities in aged specimens of cholesterol resulting in the isolation of 25-hydroxycholesterol in amounts approximately proportional to the age of the specimen. Two mechanisms of cholesterol autoxidation are summarized in figure 1.

Occurrence of Oxidation Products of Cholesterol in Foods

The earliest discovery of an oxidation product of cholesterol from a natural source was reported by *Wintersteiner and Ritzman* [16] in 1940; they found 7β-hydroxycholesterol in pregnant mare's serum. *Fieser* [17, 18] was the first to report that powdered egg yolk, the raw material used in many convenience foods, was found to contain cholestane-3β,5α,6β-triol. Later, *Pennock* et al. [19] found cholesta-3,5-diene-7-one in an avian embryo. Other investigators [20–22] also demonstrated oxidation products of cholesterol including 7-hydroxycholesterol, 7-ketocholesterol, 5,6-epoxycholesterol and cholestane-3β,5α,6β-triol in various forms of treated eggs such as spray-dried and heat-dried. Most recently, *Naber and Biggert* [23], using high performance liquid chromatography, demonstrated 5 polar oxidation derivatives of cholesterol by heating egg yolk; 3 of these cochromatograph with 7-keto-, 7-hydroxy- and 25-hydroxycholesterol. Dairy products have also been demonstrated to be the source of some oxidation products of cholesterol, such as cholest-4-en-3-one and cholesta-3,5-dien-7-one in powdered milk [24, 25], cholest-7-en-3-one in butterfat [26] and cholest-3,5-diene in butter oil [27]. Other food products such as pork fat were found to have 7-ketocholesterol [28] and beef also contained cholesta-3,4-dien-7-one [29]. Recently, by employing gas chromatography, we have surveyed some cholesterol-containing food items commonly consumed in the USA and have been able to demonstrate 25-hydroxycholesterol in powdered custard mix, pancake flour, lard and provolone, cholestane-3β,5α,6β-triol in pancake flour, parmesan cheese and lard, 7-ketocholesterol in custard mix, pancake flour and powdered milk and 7α- and 7β-hydroxycholesterol in pancake flour, parmesan cheese, lard, provolone and powdered milk [30].

Occurrence of Oxidation Products of Cholesterol in Tissues

Oxidation products of cholesterol have been isolated from both normal and diseased tissues.

Normal Tissues

Some oxidation derivatives that have been identified in the body are important intermediates in the metabolism of cholesterol. In the liver, the major oxidation derivative identified is the 7α-hydroxycholesterol which is the major substrate in bile acid biosynthesis. It can be further oxidized by specific enzymes, with addition of hydroxyl groups to the 12 position and saturation of the double bond forming 5β-cholestane-3α,7α,12α-triol and eventually forming bile acid. In the adrenal, 20α-hydroxycholesterol is a major intermediate in steroid biosynthesis which may involve other intermediates such as 20α,22-dihydroxycholesterol and 17,20α-dihydroxycholesterol [31]. In human brain significant amounts of 24-hydroxycholesterol and 26-hydroxycholesterol have been identified but their functional role is unknown [32, 33]. The 24-hydroxycholesterol in the brain is about 25–

60 μg/g dried tissue which is 10-fold higher than 26-hydroxycholesterol. Interestingly, 26-hydroxycholesterol has also been found in human aorta and the amount of accumulation appears to have a direct correlation with the severity of atherosclerosis [34, 35]. Furthermore, 26-hydroxycholesterol has not yet been detected in species other than man. The presence of cholesterol oxidation derivatives in the newborn was suggested by *Ebertein* [36] who identified four sterols in umbilical cord blood which were 22-hydroxycholesterol, 25-hydroxycholesterol, 22-ketocholesterol and 5-cholesten-3β,20α,22-triol. The presence of 7β-hydroxycholesterol in pregnant mare's serum [16] was mentioned previously and 5,6-epoxycholesterol was reported in human serum [37].

Diseased Tissue

The atheromata of human aorta have been extensively studied. A companion of cholesterol, 5α-cholestan-3β-ol, was first identified in the acetone-soluble lipids from an atheromatous aorta in 1942 [38]. Oxidation derivatives of cholesterol, including 7α-hydroxycholesterol, cholestane-3β,5α,6β-triol, cholesta-3,5-dien-7-one and cholesta-4,6-dien-3-one, were demonstrated in the arteriosclerotic aorta as early as 1943 [39]. Cholesta-3,4-dien-7-one as well as 7-keto-cholesterol were also shown in human atherosclerotic aorta by *Kantiengar and Morton* [40]. Additional major oxidation products, such as 25-hydroxycholesterol and 7β-hydroxycholesterol were found to be present in atheromatous human arteries by *Henderson* and co-workers [41, 42] using a histochemical and chromatographic technique. Also, 24-hydroxycholesterol [43, 44] and 26-hydroxycholesterol [45, 46], which have been identified in the human brain, were identified in human atheromatous plaques. *Smith and Van Lier* [34] and *Van Lier and Smith* [47] have found a total of twelve oxidation products of cholesterol in human atheromata. Other abnormal tissues which were shown to contain cholesterol oxidation products include the preputial gland tumor of the mouse [48] and both human and hairless mouse skin with formation of 5,6-epoxycholesterol after exposure to ultraviolet light [49].

Effect on Cholesterol Biosynthesis

The most striking biological effect of the oxidation products of cholesterol is their inhibitory effect on the activity of 3-hydroxy-3-methylglutaryl (HMG) CoA reductase, a role-limiting enzyme for cholesterol biosynthesis.

In fact, it is in the realm of monolayer culture of individual cell lines that recent progress has been made and has evoked great interest. In 1973, *Kandutsch and Chen* [48] reported the inhibition of cholesterol biosynthesis and HMG CoA reductase activity on cultured mouse liver cells when A, B-ring oxidation products were present in the culture medium. They also suggested the presence of more inhibitors in the mother liquor during recrystallization of cholesterol. Further studies [50] on side chain oxidation products showed similar effects. The most potent inhibitor was found to be 25-hydroxycholesterol. The functional requirements of the oxidation products suggested by this group [51] are that all of the compounds are derived from cholestane with the introduction of one functional group, either a ketone or hydroxyl at position 3, and a second functional group (ketone or hydroxyl) in the 6, 7, 15, 20, 22, 24 or 25 positions. The nuclear double bond is not required, but the complete 8-carbon side chain is necessary for maximal activity [50]. Similar effects of the oxidation products on HMG CoA reductase activity and cholesterol biosynthesis were reported in cultured human fibroblasts by *Brown and Goldstein* [52] in cultured hepatoma cells by *Bell* et al. [53] and *Zander* et al. [54] and in cultured rabbits' aortic smooth muscle cells by *Peng* et al. [55]. The subsequent effect following the suppression of cholesterol biosynthesis by 25-hydroxycholesterol or 7-ketocholesterol is the retardation of the growth of cultured cells which has been demonstrated in human fibroblasts [56], mouse L cells [57], rat myogenic cells [58], and Chinese hamster ovary cells [59]. In mouse L cells, where desmosterol is the predominant sterol, added desmosterol blocks the inhibitory effects of oxidized sterols on growth. In cultured human fibroblasts added exogenous cholesterol or low density lipoproteins (LDL) – but not high density lipoproteins (HDL) – likewise overcomes the inhibition of growth by 7-ketocholesterol. The inhibitory effects of cholesterol oxidation products on cholesterol biosynthesis and all growth also involve a diminution of deoxyribonucleic acid (DNA) biosynthesis. In mouse L cells treated with 25-hydroxycholesterol, DNA biosynthesis declined progressively and ultimately ceased. Protein biosynthesis decreased, as did growth, apparently as a consequence of diminished DNA biosynthesis and not by direct inhibition of protein biosynthesis or of other vital cellular metabolic processes. These effects can be and are reversed by addition of mevalonate or cholesterol and may be attributable to suppressed cholesterol biosynthesis [60]. Suppression of DNA biosynthesis and associated lymphoblastic transformations are also observed in mitogen-stimulated mouse lymphocytes treated with the 25-hydroxycholesterol [61] and in stimulated human lymphocytes treated with the 20α-hydroxycholesterol, 25-hydroxycholesterol and other oxidized sterols [62–64]. These effects are partially reversed by exogenous cholesterol or by mevalonate [64].

The inhibitory effects of these cholesterol oxidation products on cholesterol biosynthesis and on cell growth are also demonstrated in vivo in mice and rats. When cholesterol and its oxidation products were fed to mice at a dosage of 0.25% for 18 h, it was found that cholesterol and many oxidation products inhibit cholesterologenesis from acetate incorporation. 25-Hydroxycholesterol, 7-ketocholesterol, 7α- and 7β-hydroxycholesterol were potent inhibitors ranging from 80 to 50% inhibition while cholestone-3β,5α,6β-triol and 20α-hydroxycholesterol were noninhibitory [61]. Long-term dietary experiments [65] suggested that different mechanism for the action of 25-hydroxycholesterol and 7-ketocholesterol. They were both active in suppressing intestinal sterol synthesis, but the duration of feeding required to achieve significant inhibition by these two sterols was different. They were noneffective in regulating liver sterol synthesis in long-term feeding studies. Both sterols caused weight loss in experimental mice. In the experiments performed on both liver slices and in intact rats, *Imai* et al. [66] showed that cholestane-3β,5α,6β-triol induced specifically a remarkable enhancement of hepatic incorporation of acetate into cholesterol. This was explained as due to the ability of cholestane-3β,5α,6β-triol to depress the absorption of cholesterol from the intestine. There was a significant increase in fecal sterol excretions.

Effect on Membrane Morphology and Functions

The effects of cholesterol on the physical state of biological membranes are complex [67–70]. Cholesterol can act to condense the area per phospholipid molecule in monolayers, the inhibition of motion of the fatty acyl chain within the outer segment of the phospholipid bilayer near the polar-apolar interface of the membrane, the increase of the width of the bilayer and the increase of perpendicular orientation of the fatty acyl chains [71]. The fluidity of the fatty acyl chains of phospholipids has been shown to be a requirement for several transport systems [70] and also of (Na^+ + K^+)-ATPase [72]. The fluidity of the acyl chain probably provides the required freedom of motion allowing proteins within membranes to undergo conformational changes and rotation and/or translocational movements associated with their activity. Cholesterol could thus have a regulatory role in these processes by controlling the fluidity of the acyl chain. Permeability studies have demonstrated that the increase of cholesterol/phospholipid ratio could result in a decrease of permeability to water [73], glucose [74] and monovalent cations [75] and an increase in electrical capacitance and resistance [75]. Partial removal of cholesterol from membranes increases the osmotic fragility and glycerol permeability. In other words, the physiological role of cholesterol could be that of a 'dampening' agent, or a stabilizing force, needed for the overall integrity of the cell plasma membrane.

There are at least two possible mechanisms by which oxidation products of cholesterol could affect the membrane composition and function. As has been mentioned in previous sections, many oxidation products of cholesterol are very potent inhibitors of the activity of the regulatory enzyme HMG CoA reductase and can limit de novo cholesterol biosynthesis. The biosynthesis of DNA and mitosis cease, and a reversible arrest of cell replication at the G1 state of the mitotic cycle is affected. Cation transport in such cells is severely compromised. Plasma membranes of the cells exposed to the oxidation products of cholesterol were found to exhibit a markedly diminished cholesterol/phospholipid ratio [76]. This altered cholesterol/phospholipid ratio could result in changes in the permeability of the cells to water and cations and eventually in a profound disturbance of membrane functions. These effects, however, could be reversed or mitigated substantially by additions of cholesterol or mevalonate. Another explanation of the effect of oxidized sterols is that because of the similarity of molecular structure of these sterols to that of cholesterol there could be substitution of certain oxidized sterols into cell membrane in place of cholesterol [76, 77]. It is conceivable that the introduction of more hydrophilic groups into biological membrane may alter the physical configuration as well as the function of cell membrane [78]. In association with the inhibition of cholesterol biosynthesis produced in cells by oxidized sterols, uptake of two such compounds, 25-hydroxycholesterol and 20α-hydroxycholesterol, has been demonstrated in mouse and human cells; 25-hydroxycholesterol was found to replace approximately 75% of the cellular cholesterol in human fibroblasts when present at a concentration of 2.5×10^{-5} *M* in the culture medium. Since the largest portion of 25-hydroxycholesterol was in the non-esterified form, one can presume that at least a part was present in the cell membrane [79]. Similarly, 20α-hydroxycholesterol was shown to comprise approximately 67% of mouse L cell cellular sterol following a 72-hour incubation in the presence of 2.5×10^{-5} *M* in the culture medium. But at this concentration, it was able to overcome the inhibition of cellular growth secondary to its blockade of cholesterol synthesis presumably due to the substitution of cholesterol by 20α-hydroxycholesterol in the cell membrane [57]. *Yachnin* et al. [78] have observed several responses in a variety of mammalian cell systems exposed to oxidized sterols. Among them were transformation of erythrocytes into echinocytes with attendant changes in osmotic fragility, inhibition of chemotaxis and migration of polymorphonuclear leukocytes, inhibition of E-rosette formation by T lymphocytes in a time- and concentration-dependent manner and suppression of an immune response in mouse spleen cells. Cholestane-3β,5α,6β-triol and cholestane-3β,5α-diol-6-one were found to be most effective on echinocytic transformation of erythrocytes and inhibition of granulocyte chemotaxis, 7α- and 7β-hydroxycholesterol and also cholestane-3β,5α-diol-6-one were more potent in inhibition of lymphocyte E-rosette formation and immunosuppression. These responses cannot be readily explained since the effects occur too rapidly for de novo cholesterol biosynthesis to be implicated. Exogenous mevalonate or cholesterol usually fail to reverse these effects. Moreover, both mature erythrocytes and polymorphonuclear leukocytes are incapable of synthesizing cholesterol. The morphological and functional changes induced in them by oxidized sterols cannot be attributed to suppression of cholesterol biosynthesis. Therefore, the most likely explanation is one of direct insertion of sterically altered more polar sterols for cholesterol in the plasma membrane. Ketone and hydroxyl substitution would introduce into the hydrophobic environment of the lipid hydrocarbon chains, polar groups which would reduce the solubility of sterol molecules among the hydrocarbon chains, as well as reduce the density of hydrocarbon-chain packing around the rigid nucleus of sterol molecules. This could add to the destabilizing effects of oxidation products of cholesterol on membrane structure which follow from steric considerations alone and could further enhance the tendency of oxidation products to cause a decrease in membrane microviscosity and fluidity. The introduction of a hydrophilic group on the sterol side chain might increase the rate of sterol membrane translocation from the outer to the inner half. As a consequence, molecules such as 25-hydroxycholesterol might be poor echinocyte formers of red blood cells. Interaction of oxidized sterols with proteins of cell membranes is also a possibility. The additional ketone and hydroxyl groups of oxidation products make the possibility that such groups might, by means of hydrogen bond formation, enhance the association of oxidation products with proteins which are at least partially inserted into the cell membrane, a very attractive concept. Analyses of enzyme activities showed that 5′-nucleotidase and alkaline phosphatase were conserved, α-mannosidase and cholesterol esterase diminished and α-glucosidase redistributed in 25-hydroxycholesterol-treated cultured aortic smooth muscle cells [76]. Membrane-bound Na^+, K^+-dependent ATPase is inhibited roughly in proportion to the extent of dehydrogenation of cholesterol of human erythrocyte ghosts with a cholesterol oxidase yielding cholest-4-en-3-one produced within the membrane [80]. The membrane-associated changes would not be expected to reverse a defect produced by insertion of membrane compatible oxidized sterols into the lipid bilayer.

Cytotoxicity

Many important biological activities are attributed to the presence of cholesterol in the cells and cell membranes. The effects of cholesterol oxidation products on cholesterol biosynthesis and cell membrane functions discussed previously could influence cell metabolism, tissue viability and might cause diseases, such as atherosclerosis. Cytotoxic effects of oxidation products of cholesterol have dominated studies of biological activities from the very early period with observation made in 1911 of the necrotizing effects on frog heart preparation by derivatives of cholesterol [81]. Later, *Biswas* et al. [82] in 1964 accumulated a large number of chemical compounds related to cholesterol, but since many were available only in milligram amounts, they excluded whole animal experiments and used tissue cultures of chicken heart explants for their first large-scale screening. Of 103 compounds tested, 36 steroids were cytotoxic when 63 μg of the materials were used per culture and 15 of these produced total inhibition of cell growth. In cases of partial inhibition, the cells frequently showed cytological changes such as swelling, increased vacuolation, predominance of round cells instead of the usual spindle-shaped cells and increase of intracellular fat. *McDougall* et al. [83] chose 9 of these compounds for further study because of their close association with cholesterol which were cholestanol, cholestane-3β,5α,6β-triol, lathosterol, 7α-hydroxycholesterol, 7β-hydroxycholesterol, 25-hydroxycholesterol, 26-hydroxycholesterol, cholest-5-en-3-one along with cholesterol which produced only minimal effects on cell growth. This time they used organ cultures of rabbit aorta and demonstrated that compounds always associated with cholesterol in tissues, i.e. cholestanol, cholestane-3β,5α,6β-triol, lathosterol and 26-hydroxycholesterol had the most marked effects on the aortic cultures. Cholesterol itself had a lesser effect on the aortic cultures and this was shown with 7β-hydroxycholesterol, 25-hydroxycholesterol and cholest-5-en-3-one; 7α-hydroxycholesterol was not toxic. Cytotoxicity of oxidation products of cholesterol on other cell lines has also been reported [57, 84, 85]. In cultured mouse L cells in which inhibition of growth and cell lysis were criteria of cytotoxicity it has been shown that 25-hydroxycholesterol was the most toxic with 20α-hydroxycholesterol, 7-ketocholesterol, 7β-hydroxycholesterol and 7α-hydroxycholesterol being cytotoxic in decreasing order of potency [57]. In studies using rat hepatoma cell cultures varying degrees of cytotoxicity among cholesterol autoxidation products were found; 7β-hydroxycholesterol was the most potent, 25-hydroxycholesterol and 7α-hydroxycholesterol were less potent [84, 85]. From experiments done in the past, these cytotoxic effects of oxidation products of cholesterol appear to vary depending upon the kind of cell line used. Due to the fact that the aortic smooth muscle cell is the most important cell involved in the initial lesion of atherosclerosis, we conducted our studies to investigate the effect of autoxidation products identified and separated from USP grade cholesterol which had been stored at room temperature in the presence of air for 5 years [86]. We also studied the cytotoxicity of 12 most common oxidation products of cholesterol which were commercially available [55]. USP grade cholesterol was dissolved in methanol and was recrystallized. After repeating the same procedure three times, the methanol mother liquor was retained and was evaporated under nitrogen until a thick syrup formed. Then the syrup was dried under vacuum. The autoxidation products of cholesterol which were concentrated in the methanol mother liquor were separated and identified by employing thin-layer chromatography and gas-liquid chromatography as shown in table I. These autoxidation products along with 12 commercially available oxidation products which were further purified by thin-layer chromatography were tested for cytotoxicity using cultured aortic smooth muscle cells of rabbits. All compounds of oxidation products were first dissolved in a small amount of ethanol then added to the culture media at a level not exceeding a concentration of 0.8% ethanol. The medium containing 10% fetal calf serum served as a solubilizing vehicle. 24 h after adding the test compounds, viability of the cells was measured in two ways: (a) to one half of each specimen, 0.1 ml of stock dye solution of 0.4% trypan blue in buffer pH 7.2 was added. The number of stained (dead) and nonstained (viable) cells in a given area were counted and the percentages of viable cells and dead cells were obtained, (b) the other half of each specimen was fixed for morphological studies including

Table I. Major autoxidation products of the concentrate from USP grade cholesterol

TLC spots R_F[1] Color[2]	Identified sterols	GLC quantitation, %	TLC fractionation
1.00 0.86 beige	solvent front cholesta-3,5-dien-7-one		VI (0.80–1.00)
0.75 magenta	cholesterol	38.0	V (0.70–0.80)
0.65 violet 0.61 blue	unidentified 5-7-hydroperoxide of cholesterol	3.8	IV (0.55–0.70)
0.50 magenta to grey blue	25-hydroxycholesterol	13.4	III (0.40–0.55)
0.44 –[3] 0.33 blue 0.27 blue	7-ketocholesterol 7β-hydroxycholesterol 7α-hydroxycholesterol	12.9 6.7	II (0.20–0.40)
0.08 yellow 0.00 brown	cholestane-3β,5α,6β-triol origin compounds	5.1	I (0.00–0.20)

[1] Mobility relative to solvent front.
[2] Color development with 50% sulfuric acid.
[3] Detected by ultraviolet light absorption.

light and electron microscopy. The degree of cytotoxicity was measured as percentage of dying and dead cells within 24 h. Viable cells were spindle-shaped cells with distinct nuclei and cytoplasm. Cells showing condensed, shrunken cytoplasm were counted as dying cells and those, small, dark, round bodies with no nuclear or cytoplasmic detail were considered dead cells. The specimens were also processed for electron microscopic examination in order to provide more detailed ultrastructural morphology. The results of bioassay of chromatography bands separated from cholesterol autoxidation products are shown in table II and the results of bioassay of purified oxidation products are shown in table III. It is our opinion that the principal toxicity of the mixture of cholesterol autoxidation products of cholesterol appears to be located at bands III and I which suggested that the most likely toxic compounds are 25-hydroxycholesterol and cholestane-3β,5α,6β-triol. These findings were further confirmed by the results of testing twelve purified oxidation products of cholesterol in which 25-hydroxycholesterol and cholestane-3β,5α,6β-triol were the most toxic; 20α-hydroxycholesterol, cholestane-3β,5α-diol-6-one and cholestane-3β-ol-6-one were

Table II. Smooth muscle cell toxicity among the fractions of the concentrate[1]

Fraction No.	Dying cells, %	Dead cells, %	Total cells counted
Concentrate of 1.0 mg used for TLC fractionation[2]			
I	8.2[3]	5.8[3]	1,212
II	6.2	3.8	795
III	34.6	36.0	696
IV	6.3	2.1	1,662
V	3.8	1.6	950
VI	3.3	1.5	1,105
Concentrate of 1.75 mg used for TLC fractionation			
I	19.9	23.4	898
II	7.1	4.9	874
III	31.8	51.7	1,015
IV	2.2	1.9	994
V	3.8	3.5	796
VI	4.1	2.0	936
Concentrate of 2.50 mg used for TLC fractionation			
I	18.5	38.4	2,369
II	7.7	6.0	681
III	38.1	54.0	2,219
IV	15.6	18.1	1,873
V	3.2	2.3	1,688
VI	2.0	1.7	1,227

[1] Cell counts done by three observers as unknowns; identity of slides revealed after counting.
[2] The concentration of each fraction can be estimated from table II.
[3] Percent of dying and dead cells represents an average of the counts of three observers.

the next most toxic; 7α- and 7β-hydroxycholesterol, 7-ketocholesterol and 4-cholesten-3-one were only mildly toxic; 3,5-cholestadien-7-one, 5,6-epoxycholesterol, cholestan-3,6-dione and pure cholesterol were innocuous at the concentration of 100 μg/ml in culture medium. The minimal concentration in culture medium of the most toxic compounds required to induce aortic smooth muscle cell death within 24 h is 5–10 μg/ml; this is approximately one two-hundredth of the usual human serum cholesterol concentration. In other words, if only 0.5% of serum cholesterol is found to be toxic oxidation contaminants which might be ingested in food containing cholesterol, the aortic smooth muscle cells could be injured within 24 h. The exact mechanisms through which these compounds inhibit cell growth

Table III. The cytotoxic effect of oxidation derivatives of cholesterol on cultured rabbits' aortic smooth muscle cells

Compounds	Concentration in culture medium, μg/ml			
	10	20	50	100
Grade of cytoxicity[1]				
25-OH cholesterol	1	2	4	4
20α-OH cholesterol	0	1	2	4
4-Cholesten-3-one	0	0	1	3
7α-OH cholesterol	0	0	1	2
7β-OH cholesterol	0	0	1	3
7-Ketocholesterol	0	0	1	3
3,5-Cholestadien-7-one	0	0	0	0
5,6-Epoxycholesterol	0	0	0	0
Cholestane-3β,5α,6β-triol	1	2	4	4
Cholestan-3β,5α-diol-6-one	0	1	2	3
Cholestan-3β-ol-6-one	0	1	2	4
Cholestan-3,6-dione	0	0	0	0
Purified cholesterol	0	0	0	0

[1] Degrees of cytotoxicity was graded as percent of dying and dead cells: (0) less than 5%; (1) 5–25%; (2) 25–50; (3) 50–75%; (4) 75–100%. Results based upon average of 5 sets of studies. Degrees of cytotoxicity were very consistent.

and eventually cause cell death is not entirely clear. Two possible mechanisms have been mentioned previously. Some oxidation products of cholesterol were shown to be able to suppress cellular cholesterol biosynthesis which is essential for membrane biogenesis and cell growth. We have also utilized the aortic smooth muscle cell culture system for the bioassay of HMG CoA reductase and cholesterol biosynthesis to correlate the cytotoxicity of oxidation products of cholesterol with their degrees of inhibition of cholesterol biosynthesis [55]. The results of HMG CoA reductase activities of the cultured cells exposed to 3 μg/ml of various oxidation products of cholesterol in culture medium are shown in table IV. Among them, 25-hydroxycholesterol was the most potent inhibitor and the purified cholesterol had only a minimal effect on HMG CoA reductase. In general, the cytotoxic effects of oxidation products appear to parallel their inhibitory effects on HMG CoA reductase. It is conceivable that depletion of cholesterol content in cells and plasma membrane due to inhibition of cholesterol biosynthesis might alter the cholesterol phospholipid ratio in cell mem-

Table IV. The effect on the activity of HMG CoA reductase by the oxidation derivatives of cholesterol

3 μg/ml of sterol in culture medium	10^{-4} μmol/min/mg protein[1]	% changes when compared with control
Control	3.12 ± 0.16	
25-OH cholesterol	0.53 ± 0.05	−83.2 ± 1.6
20α-OH cholesterol	0.52 ± 0.05	−83.2 ± 1.6
4-Cholestan-3-one	2.41 ± 0.21	−22.8 ± 6.8
7α-OH cholesterol	1.27 ± 0.20	−59.4 ± 6.5
7β-OH cholesterol	1.55 ± 0.15	−50.5 ± 4.8
7-Ketocholesterol	0.68 ± 0.08	−78.1 ± 2.6
3,5-Cholestadien-7-one	3.59 ± 0.23	+15.1 ± 7.5
5,6-Epoxycholesterol	1.41 ± 0.04	−55.0 ± 1.2
Cholestane-3β,5α,6β-triol	1.14 ± 0.13	−63.4 ± 4.3
Cholestan-3β,5α-diol-6-one	1.65 ± 0.22	−47.2 ± 7.0
Cholestan-3β-ol-6-one	0.68 ± 0.10	−78.3 ± 3.2
Cholestan-3,6-one	0.88 ± 0.17	−71.8 ± 5.5
Purified cholesterol	2.57 ± 0.09	−12.0 ± 3.0

[1] HMG CoA reductase activity was determined by amounts of mevalonate formed. The data shown are averages of 4 experiments (mean ± SEM).

branes and change their fluidity, fragility and permeability and, consequently, cause membrane dysfunction and cell death. Cholestane-3β,5α,6β-triol was also shown to have remarkable cytotoxic effects on the aortic smooth muscle cells, but it only moderately inhibits cholesterol biosynthesis. An alternative explanation could be its direct effect on the membrane by replacing cholesterol in the membrane. The stronger polar groups of cholestane-3β,5α,6β-triol on the one end of the molecule and the hydrophobic groups on the other end might make it possible for this molecule to get into the membrane more easily and thereby cause profound cell membrane dysfunction. In fact, toxic effects of cholestane-3β,5α,6β-triol along with cholestane-3β,5α-diol-6-one appeared much earlier than those of side chain oxidation products. *Yachnin* et al. [78] also showed that these two compounds were most effective on echinocytic transformation of red blood cells and inhibition of granulocyte chemotaxis and postulated that insertion of oxidized sterols into the membrane is the most likely mechanism. It is very possible that through a combination of the above-mentioned mechanisms and probably also other mechanisms, the oxidation products of cholesterol are injurious to cells, particularly in arterial tissues which are constantly and maximally exposed to all the chemical compounds in the blood stream. The issue of atherogenicity probably is one of the most important ramifications of cytotoxicity of oxidation products of cholesterol; i.e. the oxidation products of cholesterol not cholesterol per se might be responsible for the initiation and promotion of atherosclerosis. The details will be discussed in the following section.

Atherogenicity

One of the most important diseases associated with cholesterol is atherosclerosis and its complications, such as heart attack and stroke. In 1948, *Chaikoff* et al. [87] induced endogenous hypercholesteremia in chickens, on a cholesterol-free diet, by subcutaneous implantation of diethylstilbestrol. In another group of chickens, comparable levels of hypercholesterolemia were induced by feeding 2% USP grade cholesterol, added to a cholesterol-free, ground grain chicken mash. After 6.5 months on these two regimens, with comparable levels of hypercholesterolemia (about 400 mg/100 ml) these two groups of chickens plus a third control group fed a cholesterol-free (ground grain mash) diet were killed and studied. Those animals eating the diet with the added 2% USP grade cholesterol had numerous, large atheromata in the thoracic aorta whereas those animals with the diethylstilbestrol-induced hypercholesterolemia and the controls both showed only meager amounts of spontaneous atherosclerosis. One of the explanations could be that diethylstilbestrol may have had a local protective effect on the arterial walls. The other possibility might be that exogenous cholesterol could contain some oxidation products which may induce more severe atherosclerosis. To investigate this possibility, USP grade cholesterol, both newly purchased and old were dissolved with analytic grade methanol and pure cholesterol was repeatedly recrystallized [88, 89]. Purity of the cholesterol residue was further assured by dibromination according to *Fieser's* [18] method. The methanol mother liquor containing the autoxidation products was retained. The methanol was evaporated under nitrogen until a thick syrup formed. The syrup was dried to constant weight under vacuum. The concentrate obtained from both newly purchased and old cholesterol appeared the same, granular and orange in color with a characteristic, rancid odor. Both the purified cholesterol and the autoxidation products were stored under nitrogen in a deep freeze to prevent further oxidation. Autoxidation products of cholesterol and purified cholesterol were given by gastric gavage in a 3% aqueous suspension of gelatin. In 24-hour short-term experiments, the experimental rabbits received either 1 g/kg of newly purchased or old (5 years) cholesterol or 250 mg/kg of the methanol concentrate of oxidation products [88, 89]. One group of controls received gelatin only by gastric gavage; another control group received 250 mg/kg of cholesterol purified by dibromination. All rabbits were killed and studied by light and electron microscopy 24 h after their single gastric gavage feeding. Blocks of tissue (1 × 2 mm) were taken from a 5-mm segment of the thoracic aorta at the level of the atrioventricular junction. Each block was oriented in such a fashion that a cross-section of the entire aortic wall was present in each section. Each section contained no adventitia; there were 18–22 musculo-elastic layers in each section. 25–30 complete transverse sections were made of each of the six blocks. One carefully selected section from each of the six blocks was used for the assay of smooth muscle cell death. The electron microscopist performed the cell counts on sections without awareness of their identity. Only portions of cell bodies with the nucleus in the section were included in the cell count so that assessment of the status of the cell would depend on both nuclear and cytoplasmic changes. The results are summarized in table V. All data were subjected to statistical analysis and indicated that the probability is less than 0.01% that the difference between the control group and the experimental groups: (a) fed 1 g/kg of old USP grade cholesterol; (b) fed 1 g/kg of new USP grade cholesterol; (c) fed 250 g/kg of concentrated autoxidation products, and (d) fed 10 mg/kg of concentrated autoxidation products, could not be due to pure chance. There was only borderline significance ($0.01 < p < 0.05$) between the control group and the group fed 250 mg/kg of cholesterol purified via dibromination as far as aggregate debris was concerned. Furthermore, the difference between the percent of degenerated cells in the controls and the group fed 250 mg/kg of new USP grade cholesterol was also of borderline significance. In long-term experiments, rabbits were given an average daily feeding of 25 mg/kg of either the autoxidized concentrate or purified cholesterol in a 3% aqueous suspension of gelatin by gastric gavage, three times per week, over a 45-day period. Those rabbits given the purified cholesterol had no lesions. Those given the autoxidized concentrate showed death of and a loss of medial smooth muscle cells with a diffuse intimal fibromuscular thickening. In this long-term study, serum levels of cholesterol, total protein, calcium and phosphorus were determined. Neither group showed deviations from normal levels.

Table V. Average frequency per 100 nucleated cells of cellular debris and degenerated aortic cells in control and experimental rabbits (means ± SEM)

Treatment	Number of animals	Percentage of aggregate debris	Percentage of degenerated cells	Average cell count per animal
Controls	15	0.03 ± 0.01	0.61 ± 0.14	498 ± 28
Old USP-grade cholesterol, 1 g/kg	5	0.70 ± 0.57*	7.60 ± 0.24**	654 ± 103
New USP-grade cholesterol, 1 g/kg	5	0.22 ± 0.08**	4.38 ± 0.54**	616 ± 22
New USP-grade cholesterol, 250 mg/kg	3	0.07 ± 0.06	1.63 ± 0.75*	439 ± 19
Cholesterol purified via dibromination, 250 mg/kg	4	1.20 ± 0.95*	0.35 ± 0.13	542 ± 95
Concentrate, 250 mg/kg	7	5.59 ± 1.99**	7.28 ± 2.86**	451 ± 47
Concentrate, 10 mg/kg	4	1.05 ± 0.38**	1.70 ± 0.67**	459 ± 68

* $0.05 > p > 0.01$; ** $p > 0.01$.

Two of the most toxic compounds in the mixture of autoxidation products identified in in vitro experiments were also studied for their angiotoxicity by intravenous administration. Injections of 5 mg/kg caused damaging effects in rabbits, including fibromuscular thickening and cell death in the aorta and segmental thickening in both major and minor branches of the pulmonary artery [90]. Of the identifiable compounds of the autoxidation products mixture used, the 25-hydroxycholesterol and cholestane-3β,5α,6β-triol were as potent as the concentrated mixture in inducing these angiotoxic effects in rabbits, the 5,6-epoxycholesterol and 7-ketocholesterol were less toxic [90, 91]. In another study, intravenous injections of the 25-hydroxycholesterol and cholestane-3β,5α,6β-triol in ethanol likewise caused aortic damage in rabbits [92]. Cholesterol purified via the dibromination did not produce damaging effects in rabbit arteries [88, 89]. By employing the scanning electron microscope the morphological changes on luminal surface of artery could be appreciated. The endothelial cells appeared to be more susceptible to the injury than smooth muscle cells since they were directly in contact with the blood stream. In this experiment [93] one group of rabbits received 2.5 mg/kg of 25-hydroxycholesterol, another group of rabbits was given the same dose of cholestane-3β,5α,6β-triol and the third group was controls given vehicle only. Both oxidized sterols were dissolved in 0.3 ml of ethanol, then added to 3 ml of the rabbit's own serum which was prepared by drawing blood before the experiment. The mixture was infused into the rabbits through a marginal ear vein by slow drip. All animals were killed 24 h after treatment and were perfused with buffered 2.5% glutaraldehyde solution via cardiac puncture for 2 h. The aortae were carefully removed and serial sections were obtained from the aortic arch, the thoracic aorta and the abdominal aorta. All specimens were prepared for scanning and transmission electron microscopy. Scanning electron microscopic examination of the luminal surfaces of aortae of control rabbits showed an undulating surface resulting from contraction of the internal elastic laminae. A few microvillous projections were seen, otherwise luminal surfaces were relatively flat elsewhere except for ovoid protrusions which represented the cytoplasm overlying nuclei. There were a few small craters, usually smaller than 0.5 μm in diameter, which were occasionally visible. Intercellular borders were discernable and the endothelial cells appeared fusiform in shape with their long axes parallel to the direction of blood flow (fig. 2). When rabbits received intravenous infusions of 2.5 mg/kg of 25-hydroxycholesterol, their aortae showed the presence of numerous blebs and balloon-like protrusions. Some of them were ruptured and formed a crater-like defect (fig. 3). Focal areas of more severely damaged aortae were occasionally seen; layers of internal elastic lamina were exposed. Other areas were extensively perforated and the surface appeared sponge-like. Many platelets, erythrocytes as well as leukocytes were adhering on or in proximity to the injured aortae. Microthrombi composed of an aggregate of platelets and erythrocytes in fibrin networks were frequently present. Some leukocytes appeared to have migrated into the subintimal space through the endothelial holes. The number of craters in ten random fields at 500 times magnification was significantly greater than that of controls as shown in table VI. The number of balloons showed only a borderline significant increase. The aortae of the rabbits given intravenous injections of cholestane-3β,5α,6β-triol showed more frequent balloon-like pro-

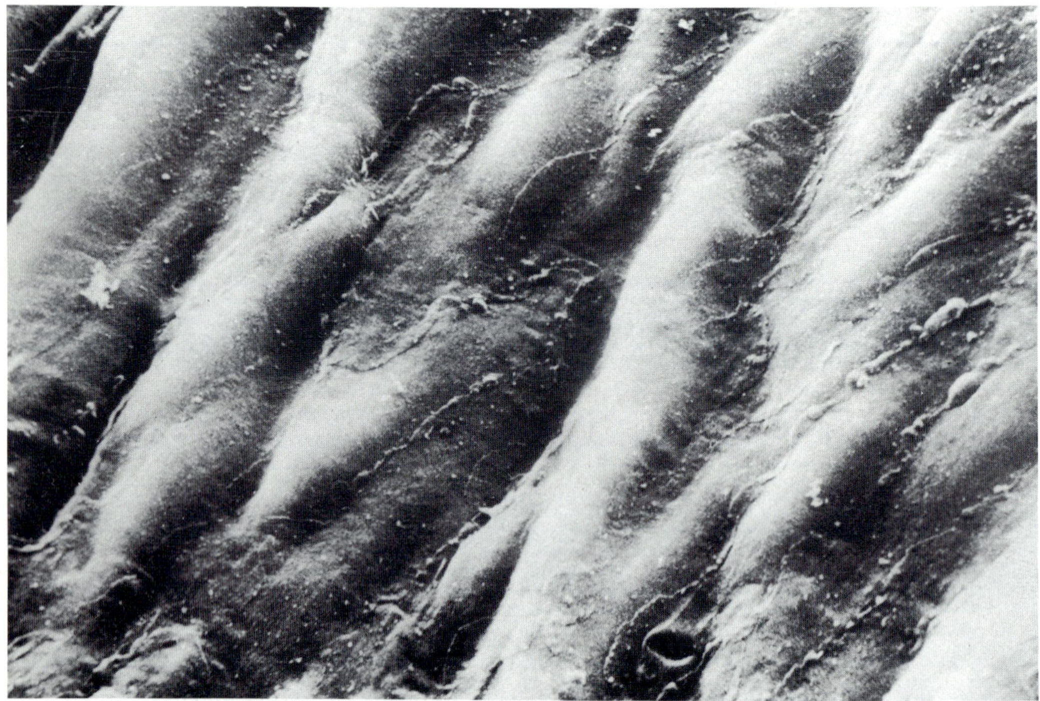

Fig. 2. Aorta of control rabbit showing undulating surface, discernible intercellular borders and ovoid protrusions of nuclei. A small crater is seen at the right lower margin. × 2,000.

trusions and crater formations on luminal surfaces which were significantly increased when compared with those of controls. Occasionally giant balloons as well as giant craters on the top of swollen endothelial cells surrounded by microthrombi were seen (fig. 4). Damage to the endothelium was also evident by the transmission electron microscopy. The aortae of rabbits given 25-hydroxycholesterol showed marked subendothelial edema (fig. 5). Some endothelial cells were almost completely detached from the internal elastic lamina. Approximately two thirds of endothelium of the 25-hydroxycholesterol group revealed some degrees of subendothelial edema or separation. Intracytoplasmic vacuoles containing edematous fluid were also seen and occasionally compressed the cytoplasm to a thin rim. Nuclear remnants and cytoplasmic debris were frequently found. Focal proliferation of myointimal cells and accumulation of collagen fibers in the subendothelial area were also evident. Rabbits' aortae of the cholestane-

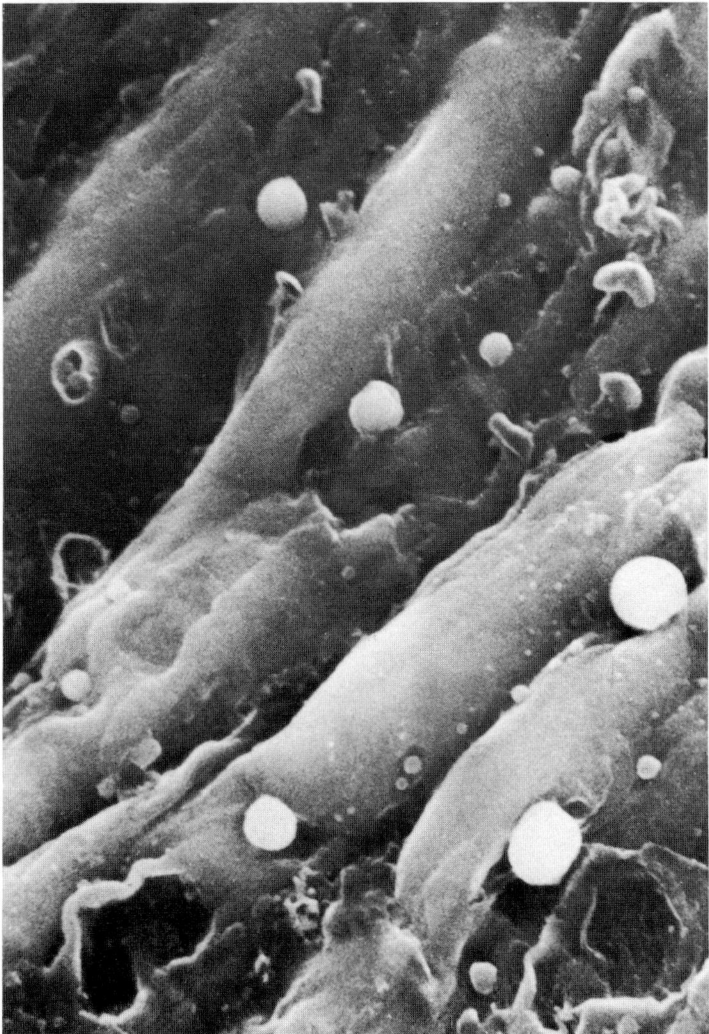

Fig. 3. Aorta of rabbit receiving cholestane-3β,5α,6±-triol showing the presence of numerous blebs and craters on the luminal surface. Many platelets are also adhering on the surface. ×4,700.

3β,5α,6β-triol group showed similar but more severe ultrastructural changes with up to 90% of the endothelium having some degrees of intracellular or subendothelial edema. Similar surface morphological changes such as balloons and craters have been described previously in the carotid

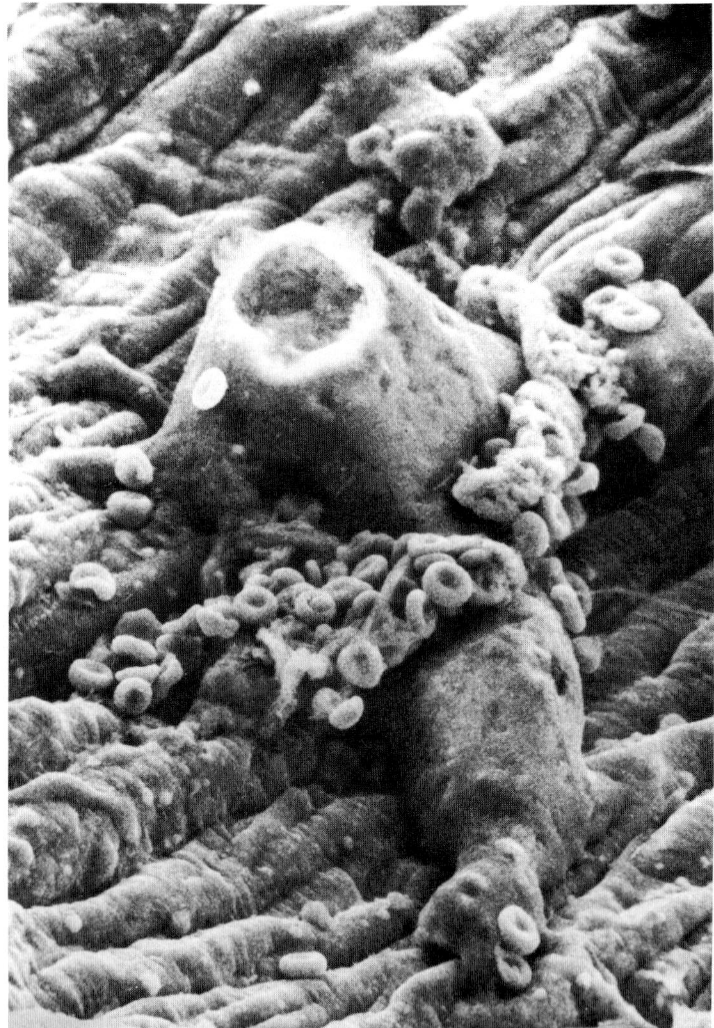

Fig. 4. Occasionally, giant balloons with conical protrusions surrounded by microthrombi and a giant crater formed on the top of swollen endothelium. ×950.

arteries of rats [94], rabbits [95, 96], and Rhesus monkeys [97] subjected to ischemia following arterial occlusions from 15 min to 2 h or aortic surface of rabbits that were maintained chronically on an atherogenic diet [98]. The sizes and frequency of the crater-like defects were found to be proportional to the duration of arterial occlusions. It would appear that balloon-like

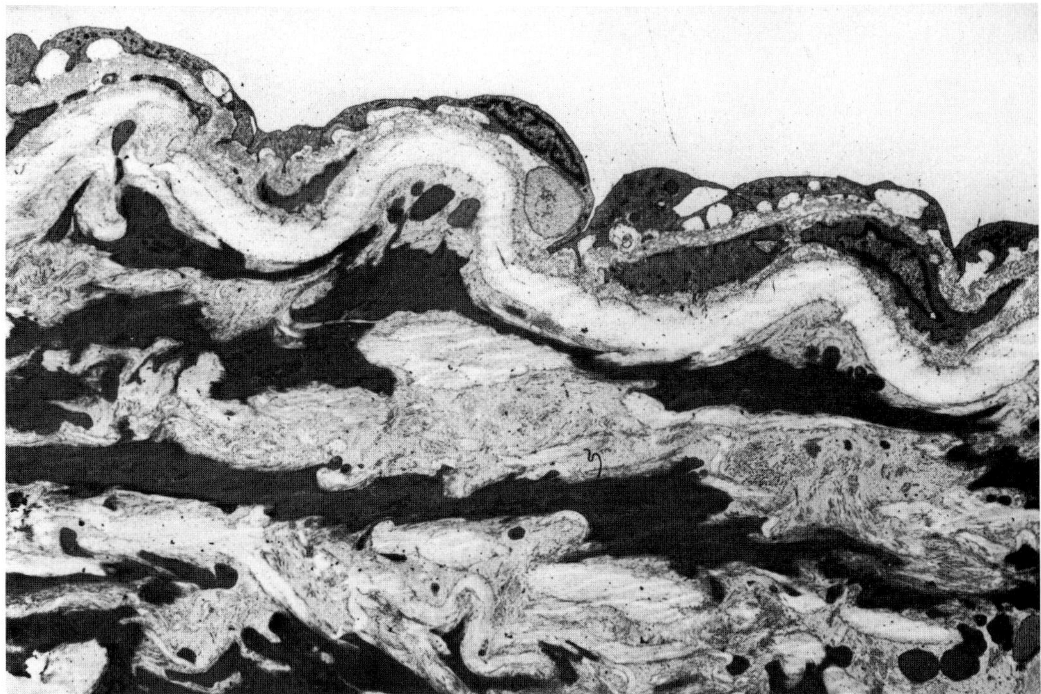

Fig. 5. TEM of aorta of rabbit receiving 25-hydroxycholesterol showing subendothelial edema and intracytoplasmic vacuoles in endothelium. × 7,100.

Table VI. Comparison of the number of craters and balloons in the aortae of 3 groups

Group	Crater	Balloon
Control	2.0 ± 0.4[1]	0.8 ± 0.3
25-OH cholesterol	6.6 ± 0.6[2]	2.2 ± 0.7[3]
Cholestane-triol	13.6 ± 1.5[2]	4.5 ± 1.3[2]

[1] Each number represents the average number ± SEM of craters or balloons larger than 5 μg in diameter for the 6 animals in ten random fields of 40,000 μm^2 (at × 500 magnification).
[2] Significant difference ($p < 0.01$) to control.
[3] Borderline significant difference ($p < 0.05$) to control.

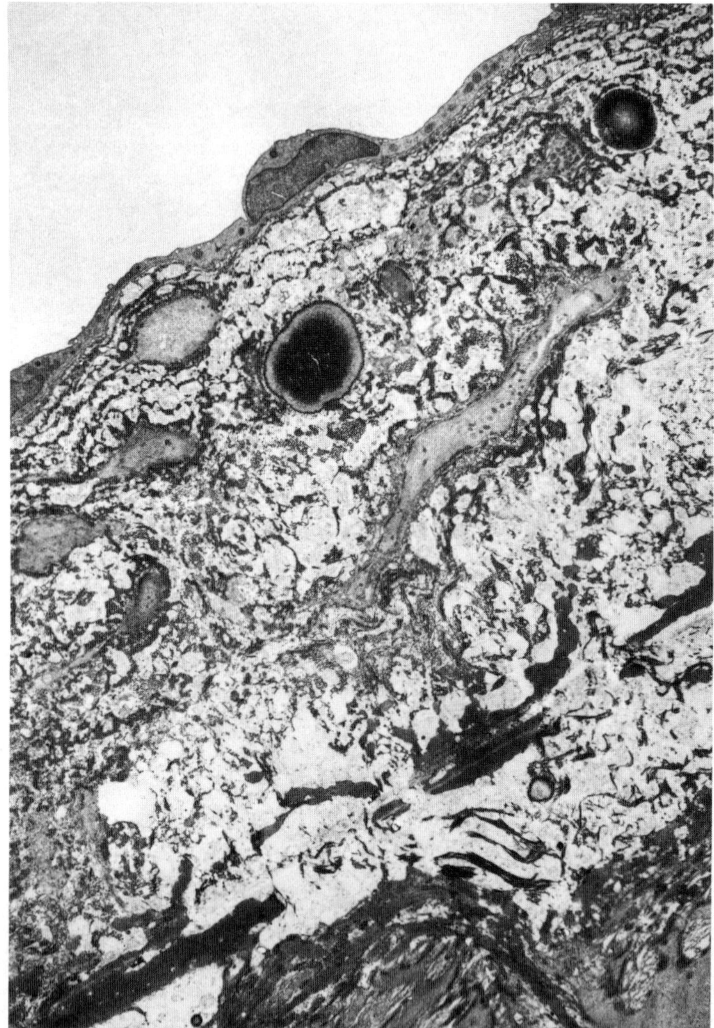

Fig. 6. Aorta of monkey fed 25-hydroxycholesterol for 4 months showing intimal thickening composed of many degenerative myointimal cells, abundant collagen fibers and scattered calcium crystals. × 5,900.

protrusions or crater-like defects are nonspecific reactions of the endothelial cells to injury. Once injury occurs, the influx of fluid containing lipids and lipoproteins would be accumulated in the subendothelial spaces [99]. Subsequently, migration of smooth muscle cells and production of collagen

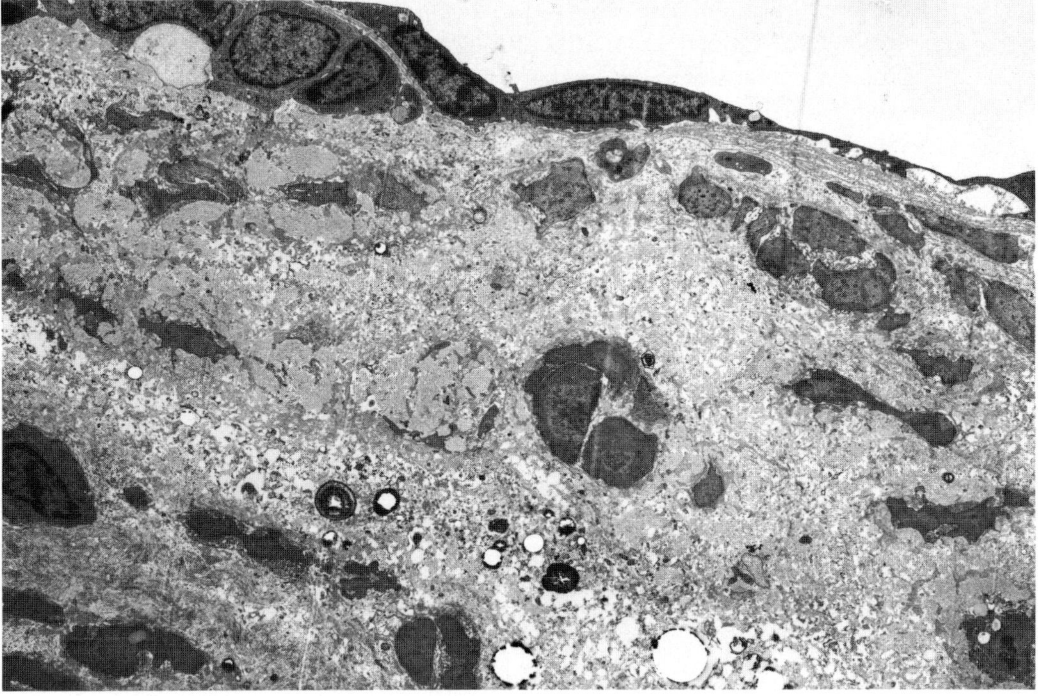

Fig. 7. Aorta of monkey fed 25-hydroxycholesterol for 8 months showing a large amount of cell debris, calcium crystals, disrupted membranes and amorphous granular materials. There are some monohistiocytes and numerous myointimal cells. × 12,000.

fibers to repair the injury and macrophages to phagocytize the excess lipids and cell debris could lead to development of myointimal plaques. In addition, numerous platelets and some microthrombi forming on or in the proximity of injured sites could further compromise the arterial lumen and aggravate the development of atherosclerosis. Recurring exposure to these injurious agents could establish vicious cycles of injury and repair and eventually the development of full-blown atherosclerosis. Long-term feeding experiments of pure oxidation products of cholesterol were first done by *Cook and MacDougal* [100]. They tested 103 compounds on organ cultures of rabbit's aorta and found cholestane-3β,5α,6β-triol to be most toxic; therefore, this compound was chosen to feed male rabbits of the New Zealand white strain with doses of 0.1% in a basal diet, corresponding to about 30 mg/kg body weight/day. The duration of feeding ranged from 27 to 350 days. Lesions were observed in the aorta, starting with deposition of sudanophilic material, graduating through various pathological changes in the tunica intima and tunica media, and terminating with the aorta showing considerable fibrosis and calcification. An 'acute' experiment, feeding cholestane-3β,5α,6β-triol at about 1 g/kg body weight/day for 5 days showed the toxic nature of the compound. More recently, *Peng* et al. [101] used squirrel monkeys which were fed 5 mg of 25-hydroxycholesterol/kg/day for 2–6 months. Arteriosclerosis induced by 25-hydroxycholesterol was visible by light microscopy as multifocal intimal thickening of the aortae. Ultrastructurally, there were evidences of arterial injury manifested as edema, degenerating endothelium and smooth muscle cells, frequent deposits of cellular detritus and calcium crystals with proliferated smooth muscle cells and macrophages in the subendothelial space, similar to those seen in human arteriosclerotic lesion (fig. 6, 7). Monkeys fed purified 0.5% cholesterol showed an increase of lipid globules and fat-laden smooth muscle cells in subendothelial spaces but no significant arterial injury. Except for these two very toxic compounds, there are no long-term studies using other pure oxidized cholesterol derivatives in the literature.

Absorption and Transportation of Oxidation Products of Cholesterol

The most important and convincing evidence needed, as far as dietary atherogenesis is concerned, is to prove 'the causative agent or agents' being absorbed through the gastrointestinal tract and transported in the blood stream to peripheral vascular tissues. There is limited information regarding the absorption of oxidation products of cholesterol. These data were derived mostly from indirect observation during studies of the hypocholesterolemic effect of oxidation products. The absorption of cholestane-3β,5α,6β-triol was reported by *Kikuchi* et al. [102] in rats and monkeys to be around 7%. When cholesterol was administered simultaneously the absorption rate could be enhanced almost 2-fold. Most of the absorbed cholestane-3β,5α,6β-triol exists as free sterol in the intestinal wall and is further transferred to the lymphatic ducts without esterification which is in agreement with the finding of *Ito* et al. [103]. *Kandutsch* et al. [65] reported that absorption of 25-hydroxycholesterol and 7-ketocholesterol in mice was about in the same order of that of cholestane-3β,5α,6β-triol. Recently, by using the dual-isotope plasma ratio technique which has been validated in old and new world monkeys by *Coray and Hayes* [104], we have been able

Table VII. Distribution of unlabeled and labeled cholesterol in various lipoproteins (all data are expressed as means ± SE)

Lipoprotein fractions	VLDL	LDL	HDL
Cholesterol conc., mg/dl	7.0±0.5	73.2±7.7	82.8±7.5
Distribution of cholesterol, %	4.3±0.3	44.9±4.7	50.8±4.6
Specific activity, dpm/mg cholesterol, $\times 10^3$	20.1±2.6	30.1±3.2	24.6±2.1
Distribution of labeled cholesterol, %	3.1±0.5	47.6±4.4	49.3±4.1

Table VIII. Comparison of the distribution of labeled 25-hydroxycholesterol with that of unlabeled cholesterol in various lipoproteins (all data are expressed as means ± SE)

Lipoprotein fractions	VLDL	LDL	HDL
Cholesterol conc., mg/dl	5.0±0.6	65.6±5.4	75.5±5.5
Distribution of cholesterol, %	3.4±0.4	44.9±3.7	51.7±3.7
Specific activity, dpm/mg cholesterol, $\times 10^3$	202±60	22.5±5.5	2.2±0.2
Distribution of labeled 25-OH cholesterol, %	34.1±2.9*	55.7±2.9**	1.2±0.5*

* Significant difference between distribution of cholesterol and that of 25-hydroxycholesterol ($p < 0.01$).
** Relatively significant ($p < 0.05$).

to demonstrate the absorption rate of 25-hydroxycholesterol to be around 30% for squirrel monkeys. Its transportation in the lipoproteins has also been studied [105]. Serum lipoproteins of squirrel monkeys fed radioactive compounds (both purified cholesterol and 25-hydroxycholesterol) were separated by ultracentrifugation into very low density lipoprotein (VLDL), LDL and HDL. The radioactivity in each lipoprotein was counted in a scintillation counter. The results showed that the distribution of labeled cholesterol in VLDL, LDL and HDL is almost identical to that of unlabeled cholesterol (table VII). On the other hand, the majority of radioactivity of 25-hydroxycholesterol was located in LDL and VLDL (55.1 and 34.7%, respectively), only 10.2% was present in HDL (table VIII). If the radioactivity of 25-hydroxycholesterol were calculated on the basis of milligrams of

Table IX. Comparison of the amount of cholesterol and 25-hydroxycholesterol in various lipoproteins (all data are expressed as means ± SE)

Lipoprotein fraction	VLDL	LDL	HDL
Apoprotein conc., mg/ml	1.07 ± 0.17	3.79 ± 0.61	28.9 ± 2.1
Specific activity of labeled cholesterol, dpm/mg protein	1,942 ± 276	8,930 ± 1,056	1,208 ± 124
Ratio of labeled cholesterol/mg protein	1.6	7.4	1
Specific activity of labeled 25-OH cholesterol, dpm/mg protein	10,400 ± 990	4,816 ± 423	116 ± 7
Ratio of labeled 25-OH cholesterol/mg protein	90	42	1

apoprotein in each lipoprotein micelle, the capacity of VLDL and LDL to carry 25-hydroxycholesterol was even greater and more significant than that of HDL (90 and 42 times, respectively) (table IX). These results showed that the majority of 25-hydroxycholesterol is transported to the peripheral vascular tissue by VLDL and LDL. The HDL carries only a minute amount of 25-hydroxycholesterol. The VLDL and LDL are, in fact, closely related and both contain β-apoprotein; the remnants of VLDL, after removing the bulk of triglycerides, are converted to LDL. The main function of LDL has been shown to deliver, to various peripheral tissues, the cholesterol needed for biogenesis of membranes and cell growth [106]. It has also been demonstrated that HDL probably transports cholesterol in a direction opposite to LDL – from peripheral tissue to the liver where catabolism takes place, and the main function of HDL is postulated to be the removal of membrane cholesterol by converting it to a nonpolar cholesterol ester through the action of lecithin cholesterol acyltransferase (LCAT). In most laboratory animals, normally, the bulk of the plasma cholesterol is carried in HDL and relatively little is present in VLDL and LDL. When animals are subjected to cholesterol feeding which is usually contaminated by autoxidation products of cholesterol, there is a substantial increase in the concentration of lipoproteins bearing the β-apoprotein. These animals, with increases in LDL and VLDL, routinely develop atheromas. Therefore, the atherogenicity of dietary cholesterol in VLDL and LDL could reasonably be the preponderant accumulation of oxidation products derived from the dietary cholesterol.

Mutagenicity and Carcinogenicity

Both atherosclerosis and cancer could be linked to the mutagenicity of cholesterol oxidation products. If pure cholesterol, which is nonmutagenic, is subjected to autoxidation by heating in air for several weeks or by irradiation for several days with ^{60}Co γ-radiation, it becomes mutagenic. The unidentified, mutagenic components were concentrated, in all cases, along with recognized cholesterol autoxidation products in the mother liquor from methanol washes. High performance liquid chromatography of the mutagenic material showed that the activity resided in the very polar fractions; thus, in regions much more polar than those occupied by the presently recognized autoxidation products of cholesterol that are chromatographically more mobile than the cholestane-3β,5α,6β-triol [107]. In the case of atherosclerosis, the suggested monoclonal character of human atherosclerotic plaques [108, 109] implies that an endogenous mutagen acting within the intima and/or media of the aorta may play a possible role in the etiology of atherosclerosis [110]. As far as carcinogenicity is concerned, the concept that mutagenic actions lead eventually to carcinogenic effects, though unproven, serves to make this a speculative concept. In fact, the original investigation of the biological implication of cholesterol oxidation products involved the possibility that some of these oxidation products are carcinogenic agents. Between 1946 and 1949 various investigators showed a high incidence of tumor development following subcutaneous injections of impure cholesterol as was summarized by *Fieser* [111]. He speculated that cholesta-5-ene-3-one was the major carcinogenic agent. Since then many oxidation products have been identified as having known carcinogenic effects. *Bischoff* and co-workers [112, 113] tested many steroid compounds including eight known oxidation products of cholesterol on Marsh-Buffalo mice. By injecting these steroids with sesame oil subcutaneously, she was able to demonstrate that five cholesterol autoxidation products: cholesta-4-ene-3,6-dione, 6β-hydroperoxy-4-cholesta-3-one, 6β-hydroperoxycholesterol, 5α-hydroperoxycholesterol and 5α,6α-epoxycholesterol were very potent carcinogens. Her results, summarized in 1969 [114], have shown that cholesta-5-ene-3-one induced spontaneous mammary tumors in Marsh-Buffalo mice when injected subcutaneously. Injection of cholesta-4-ene-3,6-dione and 6β-hydroperoxy-4-cholesten-3-one induced local fibrosarcomas. The corresponding 6β-hydroperoxycholesterol is also regarded as highly carcinogenic. The 5α-hydroperoxycholesterol was shown to provoke tumors in female mice at incidences considerably greater than in male mice, as well as in controls. However, various later qualifications, reinterpretations and assessments of other data leave these findings unsettled. A stronger case has been made for carcinogenicity of injected 5α,6α-epoxycholesterol, but *Fioriti* et al. [115, 116] could not demonstrate the carcinogenicity of this epoxide when administered in the diet. Circumstantial evidence does implicate the 5α,6α-epoxide as a putative carcinogen which appears to be formed in human [117] and hairless mouse [118, 119] skin subjected to ultraviolet light irradiation, a treatment that leads in hairless mice to squamous cell carcinoma. Moreover, antioxidants retard these events [120, 121]. *Chan and Black* [49] suggested that the potent carcinogenic effect of 5α,6α-epoxide could be regulated by the cholesterol-5α,6α-epoxide hydrase of the skin. Furthermore, the 5α,6α-epoxide induces chromosome aberrations, chromatid breaks or deletions, and initiation of DNA repair synthesis in cultured human fibroblasts; these damaging effects are like those caused by ultraviolet light irradiation [122]. The apparent covalent binding of the 5α,6α-epoxide with DNA [123] may be of further interest in this mechanism.

Concluding Remarks

Atherosclerosis induced by feeding cholesterol or cholesterol-containing foods is one of the most commonly used experimental models. Recently, it has been observed that cholesterol is quite unstable and easily autoxidized when stored in air at room temperature. The more frequently occurring oxidation products include 25-hydroxycholesterol, cholestane-3β,5α,6β-triol, 5α,6α-epoxycholesterol, 7α- and 7β-hydroxycholesterol and 7-ketocholesterol. In the past, we demonstrated that the concentrate of autoxidation products from old USP-grade cholesterol, powdered eggs and powdered milk, by recrystallizing the pure cholesterol from a methanol solution and retaining the mother liquor, when given by gastric gavage at 250 mg/kg to rabbits, significantly increased the number of dead aortic smooth muscle cells. The autoxidation products of cholesterol which were concentrated in the methanol mother liquor were separated and identified by using thin-layer chromatography and gas-liquid chromatography. In in vitro studies employing cultured aortic smooth muscle cells, these autoxidation products of cholesterol killed the cells within 24 h at an extremely low concentration, less than 10 μg/ml in the medium, equivalent to one two-hundredth of the average serum cholesterol level of humans in developed, industrialized countries. Cholestane-3β,5α,6β-triol and 25-hydroxycholesterol were shown to be the most toxic compounds. On the other hand, cholesterol, purified by dibromination showed no harmful effects in both in vivo and in vitro studies. Using scanning electron microscopy, we have also been able to show that both 25-hydroxycholesterol and cholestane-3β,5α,6β-triol produce balloon and crater-like defects in the arterial intimal surface followed by adhesion of platelets, red blood cells, white blood cells and formed microthrombi. These findings mimic the initial events of atherogenesis and these compounds probably are responsible for the atherogenicity of the 'old' USP-grade cholesterol. Separation of lipoproteins in monkeys, after feeding of radioactive 25-hydroxycholesterol, showed that the majority of oxidation products are transported by VLDL and LDL, and very little by HDL. Therefore, the atherogenicity of dietary cholesterol in VLDL and LDL could reasonably be the preponderant accumulation of autoxidation products derived from the dietary cholesterol in these two lipoproteins. Further studies on the effect of long-term feeding of a pure autoxidation product of cholesterol (i.e. 25-hydroxycholesterol) to squirrel monkeys have shown multifocal, intimal thickening of the aortae with proliferated smooth muscle cells and macrophages in the subendothelial space. Ultrastructurally, there were evidences of arterial injury and necrosis manifested as edema degenerating endothelial and smooth muscle cells, frequent deposits of cellular detritus and calcium crystals similar to changes seen in human arteriosclerotic lesions. The mechanisms of cell injury by oxidation products of cholesterol could be due either to their potent inhibition of cholesterol biosynthesis or the replacement of cholesterol in the cell membrane. Either could result in depletion of cholesterol needed for biogenesis of membrane and cell growth and also might decrease the cholesterol and phospholipid ratio and disturb cell membrane structure and function and eventually lead to cell death. We have analyzed a number of commonly consumed food products, such as a powdered custard mix, a pancake mix, cheeses kept at room temperature, lard used for several weeks to fry potatoes and concentrated infant milk formulas. All of them contain various amounts of commonly recognized autoxidation products of cholesterol. The significance of these studies appears to be a better understanding of dietary risk factors in atherogenesis. An extensive educational program to encourage commercial food producers and processors to develop methods for better preparation and storage of cholesterol-containing foods should markedly reduce and hopefully eliminate formation of autoxidation products of cholesterol in these foods.

References

1 Anitschkow, N.: Über die Veränderungen der Kaninchenaorta bei experimenteller Cholesterinsteatose. Beitr. path. Anat. allg. Pathol. *56:* 379–404 (1913).

2 Schulze, E.; Winterstein, E.: Über das Verhalten des Cholesterins gegen das Licht. Physiol. Chem. *43:* 316–319 (1904).

3 Beckwith, A.L.J.: The oxidation of crystalline cholesterol. Proc. chem. Soc. 194–195 (July 1958).

4 Fioriti, J.A.; Sims, R.J.: Autoxidation products of cholesterol. J. Am. Oil Chem. Soc. *44:* 221–224 (1967).

5 Horvath, C.: Quantitative determination of cholesterol in autoxidation mixtures by thin layer chromatography. J. Chromatogr., biomed. Appl. *22:* 52–59 (1966).

6 Van Lier, J.E.; Smith, L.L.: Sterol metabolism. XI. Thermal decomposition of some cholesterol hydroperoxides. Steroids *15:* 485–503 (1970).

7 Rosenheim, O.; Thomas, A.W.: The anti-rachitic properties of irradiated sterols. Biochem. J. *20:* 537–544 (1926).

8 Shear, M.J.; Kramer, B.: Fractionation of irradiated cholesterol. I. Chemical observation. J. biol. Chem. *71:* 213–220 (1926).

9 Dauben, W.G.; Payot, P.H.: Radiation-induced oxidation of cholesterol. J. Am. Chem. Soc. *78:* 5657–5660 (1956).

10 Bergstrom, S.; Samuelsson, B.: The autoxidation of cholesterol; in Lundberg, Autoxidation and antioxidant, vol. I, pp. 235–248 (Interscience Publ. Div. of Wiley & Sons, New York 1961).

11 Smith, L.L.; Matthews, W.S.; Price, J.C.; Bachman, R.C.; Reynolds, B.: Thin layer chromatographic examination of cholesterol autoxidation. J. Chromatogr., biomed. Appl. *27:* 187–205 (1967).

12 Van Lier, J.E.; Smith, L.L.: Autoxidation of cholesterol via hydroperoxide intermediates. J. org. Chem. *35:* 2627–2632 (1970).

13 Lythgoe, B.; Trippet, S.: Allylic rearrangement of an α,β-unsaturated hydroperoxide. J. chem. Soc. 471–472 (January 1959).

14 Smith, L.L.: The autoxidation of cholesterol; in Simic, Karel, Autoxidation in food and biological systems, pp. 119–132 (Plenum Press, New York 1980).

15 Fieser, L.F.; Huang, W.Y.; Bhattacharya, B.K.: Cholesterol and companions. X. The diol function. J. org. Chem. *22:* 1380–1384 (1957).

16 Wintersteiner, O.; Ritzman, J.R.: The isolation of 7(β)-hydroxycholesterol from the serum of pregnant mares. Biol. Chem. *136:* 697–708 (1940).

17 Fieser, L.F.: Cholesterol and companions. III. Cholestanol, lathosterol and ketone 104. J. Am. Chem. Soc. *75:* 4395–4403 (1953).

18 Fieser, L.F.: Cholesterol and companions. IV. Steroid dibromides. J. Am. Chem. Soc. *75:* 5421–5422 (1953).

19 Pennock, I.F.; Gertrude, N.; Mahler, H.R.: Biochemical studies on the developing avian embryo. Biochem. J. *85:* 530–537 (1962).

20 Acker, L.; Greve, H.: Über die Photoxydation des Cholesterins in eihaltigen Lebensmitteln. FetteSeifenAnstr.-Mittel *65:* 1009–1012 (1963).

21 Chicoye, E.; Powrie, W.D.; Fennema, O.: Photoxidation of cholesterol in spray-dried egg yolk upon irradiation. J. Food Sci. *33:* 581–587 (1968).

22 Tsai, L.S.; Hudson, C.A.; Ijichi, K.; Meehan, J.J.: Quantitation of cholesterol β-oxide

in eggs by gas chromatography and high performance liquid chromatography. J. Am. Oil Chem. Soc. *56:* 185A (1979).

23 Naber, E.C.; Biggert, M.D.: Cholesterol oxidation products in fresh and heat-treated egg yolk lipid. Fed. Proc. *33:* 581 (1982).

24 Flanagan, V.P.; Ferretti, A.; Schwartz, D.P.; Ruth, J.M.: Characterization of two steroidal ketones and two isoprenoid alcohols in dairy products. J. Lipid Res. *16:* 97 (1975).

25 Flanagan, V.P.; Ferretti, A.: Characterization of two steroidal olefins in nonfat dry milk. Lipids *9:* 471 (1974).

26 Parks, O.W.; Schwartz, D.P.; Keeney, M.; Damico, J.N.: Isolation of Δ^7-cholesten-3-one from butterfat. Nature, Lond. *210:* 417 (1966).

27 Roderbourg, H.; Kuzdzal-Savoice, S.: The hydrocarbons of anhydrous butterfat; influence of technological treatments. J. Am. Oil Chem. Soc. *56:* 485 (1975).

28 Williams, L.D.; Pearson, A.M.: Unsaponifiable fraction of pork fat as related to boar odor. J. agric. Fd Chem. *13:* 1573 (1965).

29 Vajdi, M.; Nawar, W.W.; Merritti, C.: Identification of radiolytic compounds from beef. J. Am. Oil Chem. Soc. *56:* 611 (1979).

30 Peng, S.K.; Taylor, C.B.: Atherogenic effect of oxidized cholesterol; in Perkin, Visek, Dietary fat and health, pp. 919–933 (Am. Oil Chemists' Society, 1982).

31 Sih, C.J.; Whitlock, H.W., Jr.: Biochemistry of steroids. Annls Res. Biochem. *37:* 661–694 (1968).

32 Lin, Y.Y.; Smith, L.L.: Sterol metabolism. XXVIII. Biosynthesis and accumulation of cholest-5-ene-3β,24-diol (cerebrosterol) in developing rat brain. Biochim. biophys. Acta *348:* 189–196 (1974).

33 Smith, L.L.; Wells, J.D.; Pandya, N.L.: Sterol metabolism. XXI. Cholest-5-ene-3β,26-diol in human brain. Tex. Rep. Biol. Med. *31:* 37–46 (1973).

34 Smith, L.L.; Van Lier, J.E.: Sterol metabolism. 9. 26-Hydroxycholesterol levels in the human aorta. Atherosclerosis *12:* 1–14 (1970).

35 Fummagalli, R.; Galli, G.; Urna, G.: Cholestanol and 26-hydroxycholesterol in normal and atherosclerotic human aorta. Life Sci. *10:* 25–33 (1971).

36 Eberlein, W.R.: Steroids and sterols in umbilical cord blood. J. clin. Endocr. Metab. *25:* 1101–1118 (1965).

37 Gray, M.F.; Lawrie, T.D.V.; Brooks, C.J.W.: Isolation and identification of cholesterol α-oxide and other minor sterols in human serum. Lipids *6:* 836–843 (1971).

38 McArthur, C.S.: The acetone-soluble lipids of the atheromatous aorta. Biochem. J. *36:* 559–570 (1942).

39 Hardegger, E.; Ruzicka, L.; Tagmann, E.: Untersuchungen über Organextrakte. Zur Kenntnis der unverseifbaren Lipoide aus arteriosklerotischen Aorten. Helv. chim. Acta *26:* 2205–2221 (1943).

40 Kantiengar, N.L.; Morton, R.A.: Cholesta-3:4-dien-7-one in human atherosclerotic aortas. Biochem. J. *60:* 25–28 (1955).

41 Henderson, A.E.; MacDougall, J.D.B.: A histochemical and chromatographic study of the lipid distribution in human arteries. Biochem. J. *57:* XXI, abstr. (1954).

42 Henderson, A.E.: A histochemical and chromatographic study of normal and atheromatous human arteries. J. Histochem. Cytochem. *4:* 153–158 (1956).

43 Jose, A.D.; Peak, H.J.: Failure of inhibition of cholesterol biosynthesis to retard atheroma. Br. Heart J. *25:* 133–136 (1963).

44 Chobanian, A.V.; Hollander, W.: Tissue distribution of cholesterol and 24-dehydrocholesterol during chronic triparanol therapy. J. Lipid Res. *6:* 37–42 (1965).

45 Steel, G.C.; Brooks, J.W.; Harland, W.A.: Squalene and 26-hydroxycholesterol in the human atheromatous plaque. Biochem. J. *99:* 51P, abstr. (1966).

46 Brooks, C.J.; Harland, W.A.; Steel, G.: Squalene, 26-hydroxycholesterol and 7-ketocholesterol in human atheromatous plaques. Biochim. biophys. Acta *125:* 620–622 (1966).

47 Van Lier, J.E.; Smith, L.L.: Sterol metabolism. 1. 26-Hydroxycholesterol in the human aorta. Biochemistry, N.Y. *6:* 3269–3278 (1967).

48 Kandutsch, A.A.; Chen, H.W.: Inhibition of sterol synthesis in cultured mouse cells by 7β-hydroxycholesterol, 7α-hydroxycholesterol and 7-ketocholesterol. J. biol. Chem. *248:* 8408–8417 (1973).

49 Chan, J.T.; Black, H.S.: Skin carcinogenesis: cholesterol-5α,6α-epoxide hydrase activity in mouse skin irradiated with ultraviolet light. Science *186:* 1216–1217 (1974).

50 Kandutsch, A.A.; Chen, H.W.: Inhibition of sterol synthesis in cultured mouse cells by cholesterol derivatives oxygenated in the side chain. J. biol. Chem. *249:* 6057–6061 (1974).

51 Chen, H.W.; Kandutsch, A.A.: Effects of cholesterol derivatives on sterol biosynthesis; in Day, Advances in experimental medicine and biology, vol. 67, pp. 405–418 (Plenum Press, New York 1976).

52 Brown, M.S.; Goldstein, J.L.: Suppression of 3-hydroxy-3-methyl-glutaryl coenzyme A reductase activity and inhibition of growth of human fibroblasts by 7-ketocholesterol. J. biol. Chem. *249:* 7306–7314 (1974).

53 Bell, J.J.; Sargeant, T.E.; Watson, J.A.: Inhibition of 3-hydroxy-3-methylglutaryl coenzyme A reductase activity in hepatoma tissue culture cell by pure cholesterol and several cholesterol derivatives. Biol. Chem. *251:* 1745–1758 (1976).

54 Zander, M.; Koch, T.; Bang, L.; Ourisson, G.; Beck, J.P.: Chemistry and biochemistry of Chinese drugs. III. Mechanism of action of hydroxylated sterols on cultured hepatoma cells. J. chem. Res. *5:* 219 (1977).

55 Peng, S.K.; Tham, P.; Taylor, C.B.; Mikkelson, B.: Cytotoxicity of cholesterol oxidation derivatives on cultured aortic smooth muscle cells and their effect on cholesterol biosynthesis. Am. J. clin. Nutr. *32:* 1033–1042 (1979).

56 Brown, M.S.; Faust, J.R.; Goldstein, J.L.: Role of the low density lipoprotein receptor in regulating the content of free and esterified cholesterol in human fibroblasts. J. clin. Invest. *55:* 783–793 (1975).

57 Chen, H.W.; Kandutsch, A.A.; Waymouth, C.: Inhibition of cell growth by oxygenated derivatives of cholesterol. Nature, Lond. *251:* 419–421 (1974).

58 Cornell, R.; Grove, G.L.; Rothblat, G.H.; Horwitz, A.F.: Lipid requirement for cell cycling. The effects of selective inhibition of lipid synthesis. Expl Cell Res. *109:* 299–307 (1977).

59 Nelson, J.A.; Czarny, M.R.; Spencer, T.A.; Limanek, J.S.; McCrae, K.R.; Chang, T.Y.: A novel inhibitor of steroid biosynthesis. J. Am. chem. Soc. *100:* 4900–4902 (1978).

60 Kandutsch, A.A.; Chen, H.W.: Consequences of blocked sterol synthesis in cultured cells. DNA synthesis and membrane composition. J. biol. Chem. *252:* 409–415 (1977).

61 Chen, H.W.; Heiniger, H.J.; Kandutsch, A.A.: Relationship between sterol synthesis and DNA synthesis in phytohemagglutinin-stimulated mouse lymphocytes. Proc. natn. Acad. Sci. USA *72:* 1950–1954 (1975).
62 Yachnin, S.: A comparison of the inhibition of human lymphocyte transformation by oxygenated sterol compound, human alpha-fetoprotein, prostaglandins and hydrocortisone. Blood *52:* suppl. 1, p. 146 (1978).
63 Yachnin, S.; Hsu, R.C.; Chung, J.; Scanu, A.M.: Modulation of lymphocyte transformation by alteration in cholesterol metabolism. Clin. Res. *27:* 514A (1979).
64 Yachnin, S.; Hsu, R.C.: Inhibition of human lymphocyte transformation by oxygenated sterol compounds. Cell. Immunol. *51:* 42–54 (1980).
65 Kandutsch, A.A.; Heiniger, H.J.; Chen, H.W.: Effects of 25-hydroxycholesterol and 7-ketocholesterol inhibitors of sterol synthesis, administered orally to mice. Biochim. biophys. Acta *486:* 260–272 (1977).
66 Imai, Y.; Kikuchi, S.; Matsuo, T.; Suzuoki, Z.; Nishikawa, K.: Biological studies of cholestane-3β,5α,6β-triol and its derivatives. 2. Effect of cholestane-3β,5α,6β-triol on the absorption, synthesis, excretion and tissue distribution of cholesterol in rats. J. Atheroscler. Res. *7:* 671–686 (1967).
67 Nes, W.R.: Role of sterols in membranes. Lipid *9:* 596–612 (1974).
68 Papahadjopoulos, D.: Cholesterol and cell membrane function: a hypothesis concerning the etiology of atherosclerosis. J. theor. Biol. *43:* 329–337 (1974).
69 Demel, R.A.; Dekruyff, B.: The function of sterols in membranes. Biochim. biophys. Acta *457:* 109–132 (1976).
70 Papahadjopoulos, D.; Cowden, M.; Kimelberg, H.: Role of cholesterol in membrane, effects on phospholipid-protein interactions, membrane permeability and enzymatic activity. Biochim. biophys. Acta *330:* 8–26 (1973).
71 Darke, A.; Finer, E.G.; Flook, A.G.; Phillips, M.C.: Nuclear magnetic resonance study of lecithin-cholesterol interaction. J. molec. Biol. *63:* 265–279 (1972).
72 Kimelberg, H.K.; Papahadjopoulos, D.: Phospholipid requirements for (Na^+, K^+)-ATPase activity: head group specificity and fatty acid fluidity. Biochim. biophys. Acta *282:* 277–292 (1972).
73 DeGier, J.; Mandersloot, J.G.; VanDeenen, L.L.M.: Lipid composition and permeability of liposomes. Biochim. biophys. Acta *150:* 666–675 (1968).
74 Demel, R.A.; Kinsky, S.C.; Kinsky, C.B.; VanDeenen, L.L.M.: Effects of temperature and cholesterol on the glucose permeability of liposomes prepared with natural and synthetic lecithins. Biochim. biophys. Acta *150:* 655–665 (1968).
75 Papahadjopoulos, D.; Nir, S.; Oki, S.: Permeability properties of phospholipid membranes: effect of cholesterol and temperature. Biochim. biophys. Acta *266:* 561–583 (1972).
76 Mill, J.T.; Mehler, M.F.; Adamany, A.M.: Effect of 25-hydroxycholesterol on disposition and turnover of membrane components in cultured aortic smooth muscle cells. Fed. Proc. *39:* 3009 (1980).
77 Bruckdorfer, K.R.; Demel, R.A.; DeGier, J.: The effect of partial replacements of membrane cholesterol by other steroids on the osmotic fragility and glycerol permeability of erythrocytes. Biochim. biophys. Acta *183:* 334–345 (1969).
78 Yachnin, S.; Strenli, R.A.; Gordon, L.I.; Hsu, R.C.: Alteration of peripheral blood cell membrane function and morphology by oxygenated sterols; a membrane insertion hypothesis. Curr. Top. Hematol. *2:* 245–271 (1979).

79 Brown, M.S.; Dana, S.E.; Goldstein, J.L.: Cholesterol ester formation in cultured human fibroblasts stimulated by oxygenated sterols. J. biol. Chem. *250:* 4025–4027 (1975).

80 Seiler, D.; Fiehn, W.: Effect of cholesterol oxidation on (CNa$^+$, K$^+$)ATPase activity of erythrocyte membranes. Experientia *32:* 849–850 (1976).

81 Flury, F.: Über die pharmakologischen Eigenschaften einiger saurer Oxydationsprodukte des Cholesterins. Arch. exp. Path. Pharmak. *66:* 221–237 (1911).

82 Biswas, S.; MacDougall, J.D.B.; Cook, R.P.: The effect of various steroids, mainly of the C27 series, on the growth of chick heart explants. Br. J. exp. Path. *45:* 13–20 (1964).

83 MacDougall, J.D.B.; Biswas, S.; Cook, R.P.: The effects of certain C_{27} steroids on organ cultures of rabbit aorta. Br. J. exp. Path. *46:* 549–553 (1965).

84 Cheng, K.P.; Nagano, H.; Bang, L.; Ourisson, G.; Beck, J.P.: Chemistry and biochemistry of Chinese drugs, isolated from the drug Bombyx cum Botryte. J. chem. Res. *5:* 217 (1977).

85 Nagano, H.; Poyser, J.P.; Cheng, K.P.; Bang, L.; Ourisson, G.: Chemistry and biochemistry of Chinese drugs. II. Hydroxylated sterols, cytotoxide towards cancerous cells: synthesis and testing. J. chem. Res. *5:* 218 (1977).

86 Peng, S.K.; Taylor, C.B.; Tham, P.; et al.: Effects of auto-oxidation products from cholesterol on aortic smooth muscle cells. An in vitro study. Archs Pathol. Lab. Med. *102:* 57–61 (1978).

87 Chaikoff, I.L.; Lindsay, S.; Lorenz, F.W.; Entenman, C.: Production of atheromatosis in the aorta of the bird by administration of diethylstilbesterol. J. exp. Med. *88:* 373–388 (1948).

88 Imai, H.; Werthessen, N.T.; Taylor, C.B.; Lee, K.T.: Angiotoxicity and arteriosclerosis due to contaminants of USP grade cholesterol. Archs Pathol. Lab. Med. *100:* 565–572 (1976).

89 Taylor, C.B.; Peng, S.K.; Werthessen, N.T.; Tham, P.; Lee, K.T.: Spontaneously occurring angiotoxic derivatives of cholesterol. Am. J. clin. Nutr. *32:* 40–57 (1979).

90 Imai, H.; Kanisawa, M.; Kojima, K.; Werthessen, N.T.: Arterial wall injury by cholesterol derivatives. Fed. Proc. *36:* 392 (1977).

91 Imai, H.; Werthessen, N.T.; Subramanyam, V.; LeQuosne, P.W.; Soloway, A.H.; Kanisawa, M.: Angiotoxicity of oxygenated sterols and possible precursors. Science *207:* 651–653 (1980).

92 Taylor, C.B.; Peng, S.K.; Hill, J.C.; Mikkelson, B.: Scanning electron microscopic study on arterial injury by oxidation products of cholesterol in rabbits. Fed. Proc. *39:* 771 (1980).

93 Peng, S.K.; Taylor, C.B.; Hill, J.C.; Safarik, J.: The effect of oxidized cholesterol on the aorta of rabbits; scanning electron microscopic observations. Proc. Electr. Microsc. Soc. Am., 40th Annual Meeting, pp. 340–341 (1982).

94 Bhawan, J.; Joris, I.; DeGirolami, U.; Majno, E.: Effect of occlusion on large vessels. I. A study of the rat carotid artery. Am. J. Path. *88:* 355–380 (1977).

95 Kawamura, J.; Gertz, S.D.; Sunago, T.; Rennels, M.L.; Nelson, E.: Scanning electron microscopic observations of the luminal surface of the rabbit common carotid artery subjected to ischemia by arterial occlusion. Stroke *5:* 765–774 (1974).

96 Gertz, S.D.; Rennel, M.C.; Forbes, M.S.: Endothelial cell damage by temporary

arterial occlusion with surgical clips. Study of the clip site by scanning and transmission electron microscopy. J. Neurosurg. *45:* 514–519 (1976).

97 Nelson, E.; Sunaga, T.; Shimamoto, T.; Kawamura, J.; Rennels, M.L.; Hebel, R.: Ischemic carotid endothelium, scanning electron microscopic studies. Archs Path. *99:* 125–131 (1975).

98 Shimamoto, T.; Sunaga, T.: The contraction and blebbing of endothelial cells accompanied by acute infiltration of plasma substances into the vessel wall and their prevention; in Shimamoto, Numano, Atherogenesis, II, pp. 3–31 (Excerpta Medica, Amsterdam 1973).

99 Constantinides, P.: Lipid deposition in injured arteries. Archs Path. *85:* 280–297 (1968).

100 Cook, R.P.; MacDougal, J.D.B.: Experimental atherosclerosis in rabbits after feeding cholestanetriol. Br. J. exp. Path. *49:* 265–271 (1968).

101 Peng, S.K.; Taylor, C.B.; Safarik, J.; Hill, J.; Mikkelson, B.: Arteriosclerosis induced by 25-hydroxycholesterol in squirrel monkeys. Fed. Proc. *41:* 452 (1982).

102 Kikuchi, S.; Imai, Y.; Ziro, S.; Matsuo, T.; Noguchi, S.: Biologic studies of cholestane-3β,5α,6β-triol and its derivatives. III. The metabolic fate and metabolites of cholestane-3β,5α,6β-triol in animals. J. Pharmac. exp. Ther. *159:* 399–408 (1968).

103 Ito, M.; Connor, W.E.; Blanchette, E.J.; Treadwell, C.R.; Vahouny, G.V.: Inhibition of lymphatic absorption of cholesterol by cholestane-3β,5α,6β-triol. J. Lipid Res. *10:* 694–702 (1969).

104 Corey, J.E.; Hayes, K.C.: Validation of the dual isotope plasma ratio technique as a measure of cholesterol absorption in old and new world monkeys. Proc. Soc. exp. Biol. Med. *148:* 842–846 (1975).

105 Peng, S.K.; Taylor, C.B.; Huang, W.Y.; Hill, J.C.; Mikkelson, B.: Distribution of 25-hydroxycholesterol in the lipoprotein and its role in atherogenesis. A study in squirrel monkeys. Atherosclerosis *41:* 395–402 (1982).

106 Havel, R.J.: Lipid and atherosclerosis. Cardiovasc. Res. Bull. *15:* 93–97 (1977).

107 Smith, L.L.; Smart, V.B.; Ansari, G.A.: Mutagenic cholesterol preparation. Mutat. Res. *68:* 23–40 (1979).

108 Benditt, E.P.; Benditt, J.M.: Evidence for a monoclonal origin of human atherosclerotic plaques. Proc. natn. Acad. Sci. USA *70:* 1753–1756 (1973).

109 Benditt, E.P.: Evidence for a monoclonal origin of human atherosclerotic plaques and some implications. Circulation *50:* 650–652 (1974).

110 Benditt, E.P.: Implications of the monoclonal character of human atherosclerotic plaques. Am. J. Path. *86:* 693–702 (1977).

111 Fieser, L.F.: Some aspects of the chemistry and biochemistry of cholesterol. Science *119:* 710–716 (1954).

112 Bischoff, F.; Lopez, G.; Rupp, J.J.; Gray, G.L.: Carcinogenic activity of cholesterol degradation products. Fed. Proc. *14:* 183–184 (1955).

113 Bischoff, F.: Carcinogenic activity of cholesterol oxidation products and sesame oil. J. natn. Cancer Inst. *19:* 977–988 (1957).

114 Bischoff, F.: Carcinogenic effects of steroids. Adv. Lipid Res. *7:* 165–244 (1969).

115 Fioriti, J.A.; Buide, N.; Sims, R.J.: Deposition of dietary epoxide in tissue of rats. Lipid *4:* 142–146 (1969).

116 Fioriti, J.A.; Kanuk, M.J.; George, M.; Sims, R.J.: Metabolic fate of epoxycholesterol in the rat. Lipid *5:* 71–75 (1970).

117 Black, H.S.; Lo, W.B.: Formation of a carcinogen in human skin irradiated with ultraviolet light. Nature, Lond. *234:* 306–308 (1971).
118 Black, H.S.; Douglas, D.R.: A model system for the evaluation of the role of cholesterol oxide in ultraviolet carcinogen. Cancer Res. *32:* 2630–2632 (1972).
119 Black, H.S.; Chan, J.T.: Etiologic related studies for ultraviolet light-mediated carcinogenesis. Oncology *33:* 119–122 (1976).
120 Black, H.S.; Chan, J.T.: Suppression of ultraviolet light-induced tumor formation by dietary antioxidant. J. invest. Derm. *65:* 412–414 (1975).
121 Lo, W.B.; Black, H.S.: Inhibition of carcinogen formation in skin irradiated with ultraviolet light. Nature, Lond. *246:* 489–491 (1973).
122 Parsons, P.G.; Goss, P.: Chromosome damage and DNA repair induced in human fibroblasts by UV and cholesterol oxide. Aust. J. exp. Biol. med. Sci. *56:* 287–296 (1978).
123 Blackburn, G.N.; Rashid, A.; Thompson, M.H.: Interaction of 5α,6α-cholesterol oxide with DNA and other nucleophiles. J. chem. Soc., chem. Commun. 420–421 (May 1979).

Shi-Kaung Peng, MD, PhD, Department of Pathology, Harbor-UCLA Medical Center, 1000 West Carson Street, Torrance, CA 90509 (USA)

Wld Rev. Nutr. Diet., vol. 44, pp. 155–184 (Karger, Basel 1984)

Part of Technological Processes in the Occurrence of Benzo[a]pyrene in Foods

J. Adrian, Catherine Billaud, M. Rabache

Chaire de Biochimie Industrielle et Agro-Alimentaire, CNAM, Paris, France

Contents

Introduction

Among the strange compounds of our diet, a large number of polycyclic aromatic hydrocarbons (PAH) occur as contaminant. Their origin is quite complex, including various sources and phenomena, such as an endogenic biosynthesis in plants and microorganisms, industrial operations, food processings (smoking) and home preparations (frying, broiling, roasting) which form PAH during the pyrolysis of organic matter. The investigations reveal that PAH are found in foods with concentrations ranging from a few to several hundred micrograms per kilogram.

PAH proceeding from industries and economic activities are an important source of pollution, mainly responsible for contamination of air, soils and waters. An environmental sample often consists of a complex mixture of more than 100 compounds, some having detrimental biological properties. Only a small number of these molecules have been recognized, identified and tested to determine toxicity.

About 20 are more or less carcinogenic in experimental conditions: the most important substances are 3,4-benzopyrene, 3,4-benzofluoranthene, 1,12-benzoperylene, 1,2-5,6-dibenzoanthracene; other components possess also a carcinogenic power, i.e. 11,12-benzofluoranthene, 1,2-benzoanthracene, chrysene, etc. [*Potthast,* 1975]. The data remain poor about the properties of the other PAH [*Lo and Sandi,* 1978].

Benzo[a]pyrene, so-called B[a]P or 3,4-benzopyrene, is ubiquitous in the environment and one of the most unsafe. For this reason, it is characteristic of the presence of carcinogen PAH. Its content is considered to be a valuable assessment of carcinogenicity of a sample, although it is reputed to have 1–10% of total toxicity of a sample [*Suess,* 1976].

B[a]P is a heavy molecule (molec. wt = 252), very hydrophobic, soluble in lipids and organic solvents (benzene, toluene, xylene, cyclohexane) and slightly soluble in alcohols. It can be easily oxidized and photooxidized when exposed to daylight or to ultraviolet (UV) rays. Therefore, oxidizability is the most important mechanism of its decomposition as well as in the biosphere and during the technological phases.

Because B[a]P is recognized as a strong carcinogen, its occurrence and that of one other PAH in the environment have received continuous attention. They have been the subject of various reviews [*Andelman and Suess,* 1970; *D'Arrigo,* 1971; *Jerina* et al., 1976; *Vadi* et al., 1976; *Gelboin* et al., 1977; *Lo and Sandi,* 1978; *Howard and Fazio,* 1980; *Bories,* 1982]. However, these reviews are chiefly concerned with environmental considerations and the toxicity aspects, and discuss only marginally the part of food technologies and preparations.

The purpose of this report is to renew the data on B[a]P in foodstuffs. This occurrence should be considered as a part of the much larger problem on its biosphere cycle: at first, for the plants, the origin of this substance will be presented as resulting from its transport from environment to crops. Secondly, for animal foodstuffs, B[a]P will be put forward as mainly originating from processing and home roastings.

Benzo[a]pyrene in the Biosphere

Mechanisms of Formation

Although very small, one of the natural sources of B[a]P in the environment seems to be an endogenous formation by the higher plants and inferior organisms. This biosynthesis has been proved by means of controlled laboratory experiments with fresh water algae *(Chlorella vulgaris)*, or bacteria *(Escherichia coli, Clostridium putride)*. Evidence of this synthesis was provided by the occurrence of B[a]P at a level of 5 µg/kg of dry material in bacterial pure culture [*Knorr and Schenk,* 1968].

Enzymic synthesis in higher plants was studied by *Graf and Diehl* [1966] which establish that the natural formation of B[a]P takes place independent of the photosynthesis intensity. Some works gave a great contribution to the observation concerning the endogenous origin of B[a]P in plants [*Mallet and Heros,* 1962; *Graf,* 1965; *Schmidt and Fritz,* 1968; *Borneff* et al., 1968; *Handcock* et al., 1970; *Shabad and Cohan,* 1972]. Some of them brought forth evidence that the foliage of trees – as well as edible vegetables – contain a level of B[a]P independent from external contamination and, particularly, of atmospheric fallout. They confirm that the formation of this component is correlated with the plant metabolism. According to *Handcock* et al. [1970], the B[a]P amounts are higher in the dormancy period than during active growth; likewise, they observe greater concentrations in control samples than in products from surroundings of traffic ways.

The theory of microorganism synthesis of B[a]P and its direct formation in higher plants would explain the presence of small amounts of carcinogen detected in various productions located quite far from industrial activities. B[a]P concentrations of 5.5 µg/kg of dry phytoplankton and of 60 µg/kg of algae harvested from Greenland coasts [*Mallet* et al., 1963] can reflect this phenomenon. In the same way, the finding of B[a]P in soil samples from SSSR forests ranging from 0.1 to 6 µg/kg is confirmed by *Shabad* et al. [1971].

Nevertheless, the biosynthesis of B[a]P by plants is refuted by several investigators – e.g. *Grimmer and Duevel* [1970], *Wagner and Siddiqi* [1971] or *Schamp and Van Wassenhove* [1972] – who express misgivings concerning the experimental conditions of previous conclusions.

However, technological operations as the pyrolytic processes and the combustion of organic matter, as well as natural phenomena (e.g. volcanic activities, open burnings of woods and forests, etc.) form B[a]P when the treatment or the phenomenon is carried out between 300 and 700 °C.

Indeed, during an incomplete combustion, pyrolysis or carbonization, each organic substance produces free radicals which can combine and rapidly generate numerous PAH, B[a]P included.

B[a]P also is formed by home-induced combustions. In brief, any smoke contains B[a]P which diffuses upon the Earth's surface. According to *Suess* [1976], the global B[a]P emission is approximately evaluated at 5,000 t per annum. The greatest fraction results from heatings and power generation using coal, petroleum, woods and other combustibles with an emission of 2,600 t; next come various open burnings and refuses which produce 1,350 t; then coke production 1,000 t. The B[a]P pollution from vehicles is estimated inferior to 1% of the total load, i.e. about 50 t. Recent investigations prove that aviation is responsible for important atmospheric pollution by B[a]P: aircraft eject enormous quantities amounting to milligrams per minute [*Shabad* et al., 1971].

The annual deposit of such a quantity – if it is quantitative – would represent 1 g of B[a]P per km^2 upon the Earth's surface. The reality differs from this theoretical value: the B[a]P falldown is incomplete and the deposition decreases as the distance from exhaust source increases. It will be concentrated very near to industrial centers, urban cities, superhighways, etc. Soil samples collected far away from pollution sources contain 0.5 mg of B[a]P per kg, while in the soils close to a motorway or an industrialized district the concentration reaches 3 mg/kg. It attains 650 mg/kg directly on the site of a soot factory. In the same way different levels of B[a]P are detected in the surroundings of an oil refinery [*Shabad* et al., 1971]: at the center of the factory, the soil samples contain up to 12 mg/kg. At 1,500 m from the refinery, the concentration decreases and gives about 0.12 mg/kg. Moreover, B[a]P can deeply enter into the soil: at a depth of 20–50 cm, concentrations remain the same.

The importance of penetration in the soil depends on a series of factors, among them the structure and the physicochemical nature of the earth. If its filtering capacity is intensive, B[a]P will easily pass through; inversely, if the soil has a low filtering power, it will accumulate B[a]P. Consequently, the sandy soils are poor in this compound whereas clays have great pollution. The market-gardening soils and the humus are also strongly polluted [*Fritz,* 1971]. Soils containing lignite and asphalte materials are the most contaminated by B[a]P, whose origin is endogenous instead of being exogenous as in previous cases [*Schamp and Van Wassenhove,* 1972].

When B[a]P leaches through upper layers of soils, or when it deposits directly on the surface waters, the aquatic environment also becomes contaminated. A small contribution results from water fallout, which about provides 7 ng of B[a]P per liter [*Woidich* et al., 1976].

The concentrations of B[a]P of running waters and fluvial sediments are closely connected to the pollution level from effluents. At 15 m from the draining of a coke plant, the river pollution is 10 μg/l; at 500 m downstream, it does not exceed 2.5 μg/l [*Fedorenko,* 1964].

In rivers, B[a]P is not in soluble form, but in a colloidal state, adsorbed on the suspended particles. A spontaneous reduction of this water pollution is made by a progressive decantation of the suspended matters. They contain between 50 and 2,000 μg of B[a]P in samples taken in lakes and rivers of West Germany [*Mallet,* 1962; *Borneff and Kunte,* 1964, 1965].

Various studies concerning the Seine river, between Paris and its estuary, illustrate the content and the deposit of B[a]P in such a medium [*Depuis,* 1960]. Immediately downstream from Paris (Bezons and Marly), mud deposit – between 0 and 6 m in depth – contains amounts of B[a]P from 0.4 to 8.5 mg/kg [*Mallet,* 1965]. The underlying layer, consisting of sand, shows only traces of contaminant, indicating that B[a]P infiltrates through the granular structure of sand into deeper layers. Thus, in those layers at a depth of 10 m, the more compact soils again enclose 50 μg of B[a]P per kg. Moreover, the fluvial B[a]P diffuses through the subsoil if the conditions are favorable, as in sandy soils. This is why adjacent periphery zones are contaminated upon a quite large size. Samples taken off at a distance of 200 m from river – in apparently unpolluted environmental areas – indicate a pollution of subsoil by an underground moving of B[a]P: in soil specimens taken at a depth of 2 m (sandy soil) the B[a]P concentration is within 700 μg/kg. The value decreases to 130 μg/kg when the sample is taken at a depth of 7 m (coarse sand) but increases again at a depth of 16 m (Marly soil). Finally, at a depth of 23 m (Marly soil again) the amount does not alter 450 μg/kg [*Mallet,* 1965].

B[a]P situated at a great depth is a negligible factor for agricultural pollution; conversely, it can constitute a potential hazard to the drinking waters. The ground waters contain 1–6 ng/l as is mentioned by *Borneff* et al. [in *Andelman and Suess,* 1970]. Will these above values – comparable to those of rain waters – be interpreted as a natural 'background' level of B[a]P contamination or as the quantity soluble in water? They also demonstrate that, after decantation and filtration in soil layers of different texture, the ground waters are strongly impoverished in their B[a]P content.

In another way, although a great proportion of B[a]P of fluvial streams vanish by a decanting mechanism, the remaining fraction is carried to river mouths and estuaries. Then coastal zones become polluted: plankton samples with 100–400 µg of B[a]P per kg are collected in French channel coasts, whereas some samples taken from Greenland coasts only contain on average a level 50 times lower [*Mallet,* in *Andelman and Suess,* 1970]. The food chain constituted with aquatic resources is, in its turn, reached by B[a]P pollution: large amounts of this PAH are detected, especially in shellfish from coasts of industrialized countries [*Mallet,* 1962]. It would be interesting to emphasize this accurate origin.

Mechanisms of Degradation

The natural decomposition of B[a]P depends on two factors which contribute to its partial disappearance in the biosphere. Firstly, the soil microorganisms *(Bacterium megaterium, Pseudomonas)* are able to concentrate and to metabolize this PAH. Series of microbial strains, cultivated in sterilized soil medium, destroy approximately 50–80% of initial B[a]P within 5 days [*Shabad* et al., 1971; *Poglazova* et al., 1966, 1972a, b]. The in situ B[a]P destruction is dependent on the conditions, favorable or not, to development of soil bacteria.

In marine medium, an analogous situation is described by *Malaney* et al. [1967], *Ilnitsky* et al. [1971], and *Reichert* et al. [1971]. Yet this latter biodegradation mechanism seems to be less important, presumably because aquatic microorganisms metabolize alkanes and aliphatic hydrocarbons to a much greater extent than the polycyclic compounds [National Academy of Science, 1975].

The persistence of large quantities of B[a]P in soil and aquatic media indicate that the enzymic degradation of B[a]P by microorganisms remains a doubtful phenomenon. For this reason, it is considered as a secondary reduction possibility. This conclusion is reinforced by some observations reported about the ability of activated sludges used for the destruction of PAH from waste water by oxidation: this class of compounds is extremely resistant to a biological oxidation [*Malaney* et al., 1967].

The second mechanism of destruction, the most significant, is the possibility of a photooxidation or a chemical oxidation in the atmosphere. B[a]P is a light- and oxygen-sensitive compound; its degradation is similarly affected by the sunlight and UV rays (near to 365 nm), as well as other oxidizing agents occurring in the atmosphere (ozone, nitrogen oxides, sulfur oxides) [*Andelman and Suess,* 1971; *Rohrlich and Suckow,* 1973; *Suess,* 1972, 1976]. This oxidation is proportional to the temperature, oxygen concentration and light intensity. For example, in solution, a daylight illumination of about 8,000 lux during 20 h is required to degrade approximately 90% of B[a]P [*Suess,* 1976]. This mechanism, jointly acting with UV rays and oxygen, can destroy B[a]P in air and in the surface of soil and waters. The oxidation becomes impossible when the oxidant factors and the rays cannot reach B[a]P situated at any depth in soils and waters.

Finally, although the true intensity of B[a]P degradation cannot be presently estimated, the two mechanisms of natural degradation are unable to destroy all the PAH emitted in the Earth's surface. Since the beginning of the 19th century, it can be concluded that the accelerated economic development of industries provokes an increase in the output of B[a]P and its progressive accumulation in the biosphere.

Benzo[a]pyrene in Foods

B[a]P is known to occur in various categories of foods; since it is carcinogenic, its origin and its level are of a considerable interest. The contamination of crops by atmospheric pollution is a frequent source of food B[a]P. Besides this origin, numerous heatings, directly or not, play an important part in the B[a]P concentration of the finished product. Conversely, some technologies provoke a notable reduction of B[a]P contained in the crude foodstuff.

PAH only appears above 250 °C. According to the chemical components of the product and when a pyrolytic mechanism occurs, the amount of PAH is directly proportional to the heating and, over a range of temperatures between 400 and 700 °C, is very important. Pyrolysis of some food constituents, such as carbohydrates and amino acids, provide any PAH, but that of lipid materials mostly contribute to the formation of these molecules. With the lipids, the PAH synthesis can be explained since they contain natural polycyclic elements, like sterols, which rapidly give PAH molecules [*Davies and Wilmshurst,* 1960; *Masuda* et al., 1967; *Halaby and Fagerson,* 1970; *Grimmer,* 1970; *Schmeltz and Hoffmann,* 1976]. Yet the temperatures used for domestic and industrial wet cookings and those of sterilizing procedures are too low to generate the B[a]P, contrarily to temperatures reached during grilling, roasting or frying. Another origin of food PAH is the smoke-curing treatment as preservation technique.

For these different reasons, the presence of B[a]P in foods is very frequent. It can be a real prejudice to the field of public health since a correlation might exist between the incidence of gastric cancer and the consump-

Table I. Evaluation of B[a]P ingestion in the GDR, per capita and per annum [from *Fritz,* 1971, 1981, 1983; *Fritz and Uhde,* 1982]

Consumed amount kg/year		Bringing in B[a]P (µg/year) by food products from: rural countries		industrialized countries
88.5	cereal products	30.1		168.2
	direct drying		60.2	
138.7	potatoes		12.5	
1.2	beans and lentils		1.0	
1.8	rice		1.3	
98.1	vegetables	44.1		598.4
40.3	fruits	8.0		92.7
19.7	exotic fruits		0.8	
1.9	vegetable fats		6.1	
10.5	margarines		27.3	
86.2	meat and derivatives			
51.7	unsmoked		7.8	
34.0	smoked		18.7	
0.5	open-fire grilled		3.2	
6.9	fish and derivatives			
5.9	unsmoked		1.1	
1.0	smoked		1.9	
	beverages			
1,000.0	water		4.4	
2.7	coffee		0.8	
0.1	tea		0.4	
130.0	beer		10.4	
Annual B[a]P ingested		179.9		957.0

tion of smoke-cured foods [*Dungal,* 1961; *Dungal and Sigurjonsson,* 1967]. Among others, the German authorities have felt the importance of this question and they have established a regulation about the B[a]P level in foods.

Concerning the GDR, the B[a]P consumption varies between 250 and 1,000 µg per annum and per capita (table I). In this evaluation, the usual plant foods (cereals, fruits and vegetables) supply between 45 and 90% of ingested B[a]P. Contrarily, the smoke-cured and roasting products always represent a very small contribution. Table I also illustrates the role of geographic origin of foodstuffs: those from industrialized countries contain 3–5 times as much B[a]P as those of rural zones.

Benzo[a]pyrene in Food Plants

The origin of B[a]P detected in plants seems to be quite ambiguous and various; it is not completely elucidated: according to several authors, a fraction of B[a]P may spring from endogenous synthesis, but there is a disagreement about its importance. For others, the preponderant way of B[a]P appearance is a pollution provided by the atmosphere, soil or water. The contamination of the leaves may occur by the deposit of dusts and soots which contain many PAH. However, when vegetable leaves are washed, only 10% of the B[a]P content disappears [*Grimmer and Hildebrandt,* 1965]. Consequently, what is an external deposit? Probably B[a]P can slightly penetrate the external tissues of plants, since studies on cereals reveal that B[a]P is focused in external fractions of plants.

B[a]P concentrations observed in straw are much higher than in grain which is less exposed to pollution of atmospheric origin [*Shabad and Cohan,* 1972]:

Kind of wheat and production year	B[a]P concentration, μg/kg		
	straw	grain	straw/grain
Saratovskaya (1969)	4.52	0.29	15.6
Erythrospernum (1970)	27.0	0.84	32.2

Likewise, the chaff of grain is more subject to B[a]P from the atmosphere than the grain itself. This is why the husking process decreases the B[a]P concentration by 60% means of elimination of 3.5–4.0% of husk [*Rohrlich and Suckow,* 1970]. Further studies will reveal that the B[a]P is located in the pericarp of the grain itself.

Proofs of this selective location are produced by other observations. Wheat irradiated by daylight shows a B[a]P decrease of about 50% within 30 days [*Rohrlich and Suckow,* 1970, 1971]. Also, a superficial localization of atmospheric B[a]P can be confirmed by means of oranges as an example: no polluant is detected in the edible parts, a solubilization of B[a]P in essential oils of the peel could explain this fact [*Gunther* et al., 1967].

If, in a simplified examination, a proportionality appears between the B[a]P content in soil and that of plants [*Fritz and Engst,* 1971], the origin of this relation can be the atmospheric contribution which pollutes both the aerial part of vegetables and the soil. Indeed, the relation soil B[a]P/plant B[a]P is loose and, generally, the B[a]P concentrations in vegetables do not necessarily reflect the pollution levels in soils [*Siegfried,* 1975a; *Siegfried and Müller,* 1978].

Nevertheless, the B[a]P contained in soil penetrates into the plant roots [*Dörr,* 1965; *Shabad,* 1968; *Shabad and Cohan,* 1972; *Siegfried,* 1975a; *Müller,* 1976; *Siegfried and Müller,* 1978]. In the case of food roots and tubers, this B[a]P mainly remains in the peel. In practice, this external location is a safety factor for the consumer since the home preparations eliminate the polluant: if the potato peelings contain 0.36 μg of B[a]P per kg, its concentration will not exceed 0.09 μg in the pulp [*Shabad and Cohan,* 1972]. Identical results are obtained with carrots: peeling excludes the three quarters of B[a]P initially held in roots [*Siegfried,* 1975a; *Siegfried and Müller,* 1978].

On several observations, levels of B[a]P appear inferior in roots than in vegetable leaves. For example, carrots contain 0.07–0.14 μg of B[a]P per kg of dry matter, whereas in lettuce the content varies from 0.20 to 1.30 μg/kg [*Siegfried,* 1975a], i.e. 10 times higher. This confirms the importance of direct pollution by the atmosphere.

Each kind of plant tends to show a more or less characteristic B[a]P level. The example below concerns vegetables cultivated in a suburb of an industrialized city [*Grimmer and Hildebrandt,* 1965]:

	Number of samples	B[a]P concentration, μg/kg	
		mean	extreme values
Salad	5	5.95	2.95–12.80
Cabbage	4	18.30	12.60–24.50

In the same series, tomatoes are strongly spared, with quantities which do not exceed 0.22 μg/kg. Such differences are attributable to facilities of B[a]P deposit on the vegetables: the slight pollution of tomatoes can result because of the small surface that they expose to atmospheric pollution. The

Table II. B[a]P concentration in vegetables according to their geographic location, in μg/kg of dry matter

Vegetable	Country of production		Author
	industrialized	rural	
Salad	12.8	2.9	*Tilgner* [1971]
Cabbage	24.5	20.5	*Tilgner* [1971]
Wheat	0.47	0.13	*Tilgner* [1971]
Wheat	2.20	0.73	*Fritz* [1971]
Wheat	0.29	0.15	*Soos* [1974]
Barley	1.12	0.30	*Soos* [1974]
Rye	0.70	0.16	*Tilgner* [1971]

large pollution of cabbage reflects its slow growth which exposes leaves to pollution during a long time.

First of all, the B[a]P detected in plants would result from a direct or indirect deposition of air particles: tissues and organs exposed to air would be contaminated according to the duration of exposure and to the ease with which B[a]P may deposit on the aerial organs of plants. The importance of this factor is indeed confirmed by comparative analysis presented in table II. According to *Kedzierski* [1975], the variations can reach a ratio of 1:10.

An analogous observation is made concerning the lead pollution of foodstuffs submitted to urban atmosphere, in external shop windows: the lead deposits are proportional to surface/weight ratios of fruits and vegetables [*Beaud* et al., 1982].

Consequently, the most probable mechanism of plant pollution is a direct deposit of atmospheric B[a]P, which remains in outside layers of vegetable tissues.

Influence of Technological Processes

Beyond the processes of grilling, roasting and smoke curing, various technologies modify, somehow, the B[a]P level of crude foodstuffs. In particular, refining and treatment in an oxidizing medium can eliminate or destroy a large fraction of B[a]P. The following examples are linked to processes or operations which have consequential effects on the B[a]P content of our diet.

Table III. B[a]P concentration in yeasts and their culture medium [from *Grimmer and Wilhelm,* 1969]

	µg/kg of dry matter
Component of culture medium	
Molasses	0.55
Bisulfitic liquor (paper by-product)	0.40
Yeasts cultivated in aerobic conditions	
Food yeast (West of France)	1.30
Baking yeast (Saxony)	1.80
Baking yeast (South of France)	8.00
Baking yeast (Paris)	12.20
Baking yeast (Hamburg)	13.20
Baking yeast (Edinburgh)	40.40
Yeast cultivated in anaerobic conditions	
Distillery yeast	0.90

Benzo[a]pyrene in Yeasts

The occurrence of this compound in yeasts rises both from technological procedures and from the nature of environment. When yeast is a by-product of alcoholic fermentation (distillery yeast, brewer's yeast), Saccharomyces strain growth is achieved in anaerobic conditions; in this case, no outside air carrying B[a]P is delivered to the fermentation medium.

On the contrary, when the aim is a production of biomass (single cell protein), a very aerobic medium is required. In these circumstances, cells come into permanent contact with a great volume of air, which may be polluted by the B[a]P. That is why yeasts grown in aerobic media contain on the average 5 times more B[a]P than the brewer's yeasts [*Morimoto* et al., 1974].

Moreover, levels of B[a]P found in aerobic yeast cultures reflect the degree of pollution neighboring a yeast factory. From the *Grimmer and Wilhelm* [1969] analysis presented in table III, the concentration of B[a]P in aerobic yeasts varies in a ratio from 1 to 31 according to industrialization degree of environment.

Concerning the British Petroleum procedures for the yeast production from a petroleum substrate, the pollution level appears very small because of characteristic operations: the crude petroleum is previously treated by molecular screening to obtain the alkane fraction, or the crude yeast cultivated on petroleum is totally relieved of its hydrocarbon residue [*Grimmer and Wilhelm,* 1969; *Takata,* 1969; *McGinnis,* 1975; *McGinnis and Norris,* 1975; *Truhaut and Ferrando,* 1976; *Santoro* et al., 1979].

Table IV. B[a]P concentration in various fat products [from the compilation of *D'Arrigo,* 1971]

	µg/kg	
	mean	extreme values
Olive oil	8.8	0.5–30.0
Coconut butter	23.1	0.7–62.0
Sunflower oil	16.1	1.0–41.0
Peanut oil	7.9	0.6–35.0
Soybean oil	2.8	1.4–6.0
Maize oil	2.9	0.7–6.0
Palm butter		4.1–6.0
Palm oil		1.2–8.0
Cotton oil		0.4–5.0
Linseed oil		1.4–3.0
Margarine		0.2–8.2
Fish oil		1.0–5.1
Butter	0[1]	

[1] B[a]P is not identified.

Benzo[a]pyrene in Fats

Every part of vegetable oils and fats contain variable concentrations of B[a]P [*Heffter,* 1970; *Siegfried,* 1975b; *D'Arrigo,* 1971]. On the other hand, butter does not seem to include B[a]P [*Le Clerc* et al., 1966; *Fabian,* 1968; *D'Arrigo,* 1971; *Prokhorova and Mironova,* 1973; *Swallow,* 1976]. Some analyses detect about 0.5 µg of B[a]P per kg of butter [*Siegfried,* 1975b; *Lintas* et al., 1979].

Does this lack mean that the mammary gland is opposed to B[a]P transfer to milk? Probably the ruminant digestive flora modifies the food PAH. Does milk perhaps contain metabolites of B[a]P and no hydrocarbon molecules? A similar explanation may be given about other animal shortenings since they are also poor in B[a]P [*Soos,* 1979].

Concerning the vegetal products (table IV), the B[a]P levels depend on the oil's nature: soybean and colza are less polluted than coconut and sunflower oils. Probably these differences are due to agronomic stage (atmospheric pollution, possibility of a B[a]P accumulation in plants and in their lipids, etc.). Indeed, no fact can establish an appreciable increase of B[a]P level during the technological stage; on the contrary, some treatments lead to an important degradation or destruction of B[a]P contained in crude oils.

First of all, solvents used for oil extraction do not constitute an additional source of B[a]P in these products, at least in correct conditions [*Tilgner,* 1970; *D'Arrigo,* 1971; *Howard* et al., 1968]. To support this statement, olive oils – which do not result from a solvent extraction procedure – are indistinguishable from other commercial oils.

Subsequent processing operations strongly determine the residual B[a]P found in refined oil. Even though during the elimination of 'mucilage' with aqueous treatment and the chemical neutralization by sodium hydroxide, the B[a]P quantities are unchanged [*Grigorenko* et al., 1971], various other refining stages are very adequate for removing the B[a]P.

Deodorization with steam under vacuum provokes some loss of B[a]P provided that steam is injected under high temperatures and duration of treatment is sufficient [*Biernoth and Rost,* 1968; *Grigorenko* et al., 1972].

To eliminate B[a]P and various other detrimental substances, blenching with activated charcoals or fuller's earth represents the most interesting phase [*Biernoth and Rost,* 1967, 1968]: treatment with 0.25% of activated charcoal was enough to reduce to 10% the B[a]P concentration of oil.

In another way, margarines are usually poor in B[a]P since the hydrogenation process provokes a destruction and an elimination of this substance [*Fabian,* 1968; *Fritz,* 1968d; *Prokhorova and Mironova,* 1973; *Prokhorova* et al., 1973]. In this case, the detected B[a]P arises from various ingredients added to the hydrogenated oil.

Benzo[a]pyrene in Cereal Products

In spite of the importance of geographical location (table II), technological operations strongly determine the amount of contaminant found in cereal products.

Firstly, at the time of harvest, when the grain requires a drying and if combustion gases are directly applied for drying, a large increase of B[a]P concentration in grain is observed. The phenomenon is very important in the case where lignite is the combustible [*Bolling,* 1964; *Rohrlich and Suckow,* 1970; *Fritz,* 1974]. The drying operations may be responsible for B[a]P levels of 7.5–10.0 µg/kg instead of 0.7–1.2 µg/kg in control samples.

Secondly, during the milling, bolting is a possibility of an important elimination, B[a]P being concentrated in outside layers of grain. Table V and figure 1 show the strict relationship between the rate of flour extraction and the B[a]P concentration in milled products.

Thirdly, the baking technology also modifies the B[a]P levels in baked and grilled products. On the one hand, oxidative mechanisms extend during

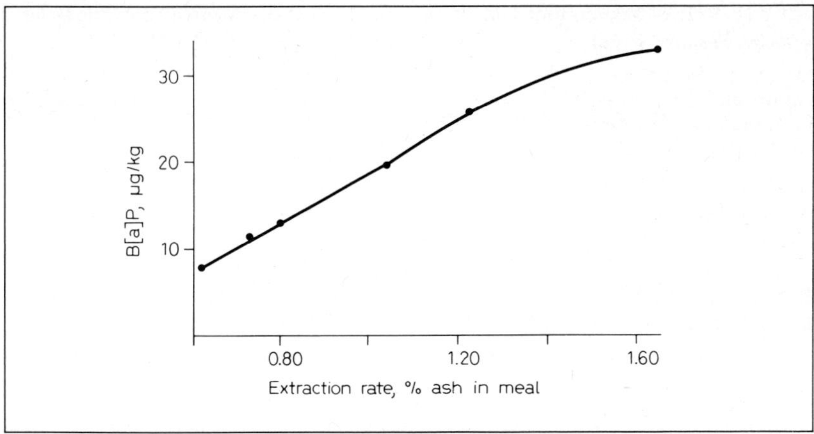

Fig. 1. Role of bolting on the B[a]P amount in flour [from *Rohrlich and Suckow,* 1971].

Table V. B[a]P concentration in milled cereal products [from *Rohrlich and Suckow,* 1971]

	B[a]P content in	
	% of grain	µg/kg
Wheat with 1.35 µg of B[a]P per kg[1]		
Patent flour	62.7	0.96
Middling bran	26.0	2.10
Coarse bran	10.3	3.44
Wheat with 26.8 µg of B[a]P per kg[1]		
Patent flour	60.0	7.4
Middling bran	22.0	38.0
Coarse bran	16.5	88.0

[1] Artificially contaminated through smoking.

the kneading and the cooking of dough (table IV): air introduced by kneading contributes to partially oxidize the B[a]P during the cooking [*Fritz,* 1968b; *Rohrlich and Suckow,* 1973]. If improving agents are added to the dough, their presence reinforces the oxidation, insofar as they act as oxidants. Bromate and iodate are immediately active. The ascorbic acid – reducing in its initial state – only becomes active by its conversion in dehy-

Table VI. Role of baking aging factors on the B[a]P loss during bread cooking [from *Rohrlich and Suckow,* 1973]

Nature and concentration of the addition to the flour	Loss of B[a]P during the baking process %
Control	20.5
Ascorbic acid (0.003%)	21.5
Ascorbic acid (0.003%) + oxidase	48.5
Ascorbic acid (0.010%) + oxidase	69.0
K bromate (0.005%)	44.0
K iodate (0.0005%)	40.5

droascorbic acid; an enzymic system facilitates this transformation. Finally, with these aging factors, at least 40% of B[a]P are destroyed in bread crumb (table VI).

On the other hand, when cereal products are exposed to grilling or toasting, temperatures used are responsible for B[a]P formation from pyrolysis of biochemical components of the product. For example, the bread crust contains more B[a]P than the crumb: 0.3–0.5 against 0.2 µg/kg inside the bread [*Fritz,* 1968b]. The amount of B[a]P in highly grilled biscuits virtually increases 2-fold compared to flour [*Fritz,* 1968b]. Toasting of bread also produces a strong increase of B[a]P concentration: 70 and 145% after 3 and 5 min of toasting, respectively [*Lintas* et al., 1979].

Benzo[a]pyrene in Drinking Water

Nowadays, there are different techniques for removal of B[a]P present in water. At first, a filtration or centrifugation operation is an initial and essential stage to eliminate the B[a]P contained in suspended solids. Next, some more or less specific processes may be used. The efficiency of crossing through activated charcoal is the same in the case of water treatment as with oil purification [*Borneff and Fischer,* 1961]. Dephenolization is also able to eliminate the B[a]P [in *Andelman and Suess,* 1970].

Other operations such as photooxidation and chemical oxidation have been tested [*Ilnitsky* et al., 1971; *Gräf and Nothhafft,* 1963]. These trials are not completely convincing. Particularly chlorine use provokes a weak oxidation.

In brief, a correct treated water should not be a perceptible cause of pollution. As long as suitable technologies are set in action, it must be easy

Table VII. B[a]P concentration in coffee, according to the roasting intensity

Author	μg of B[a]P per kg of roasted coffee		
	weak roasting	middle roasting	strong roasting
Malanoski et al. [1968]	0	–	–
Soos and Följy [1974]	–	0.8–6.0	–
IARC [1973]	–	–	15.0
Fritz [1968a]	–	0.3–0.5	–
Kuratsune and Hueper [1960]	0	–	0–4.0

to reach the B[a]P concentrations of ground waters, i.e. from 1 to 6 ng/l, even from a surface water which is highly contaminated.

Benzo[a]pyrene in Roasted Products

Intensive heat treatments – made by industry or at home – lead to the production of B[a]P. Coffee has been studied by different authors because of the heat intensity used for its roasting. According to the analysis presented in table VII, the B[a]P concentrations in roasted beans are very low and even zero. Yet, the concentrations appear slightly proportional with the duration and intensity of roasting: the American coffees are practically devoid of B[a]P, the Italian products usually contain small quantities.

It is worth noting that the B[a]P levels in green and roasted coffee oils are the same [*Bracco,* 1973]. Nevertheless, the formation of B[a]P during the roasting is obvious: the roaster tars can contain 245 μg of B[a]P per kg [*Fritz,* 1975] and the soots between 200 and 400 μg [*Kuratsune and Hueper,* 1958]. Thus, probably, the greatest quantity of formed B[a]P vanishes in the atmosphere during the operation.

The remaining fraction easily passes into the coffee which is drunk, the coffee grounds being poor in B[a]P. According to *Fritz* [1969], caffeine favors the solubilization of B[a]P in boiling water.

Instant coffees contain little or no B[a]P [*Kuratsune and Hueper,* 1960; *Bracco,* 1973; *Strobel,* 1974; *Soos and Fözy,* 1974]. Drinkings made from bean coffee or soluble powder provide a comparable content of B[a]P; this is estimated at approximately 0.1 ng per coffee cup.

The broiling of meats on an open fire also shows a PAH formation with respect to well-known practices and mechanisms: (1) The lipid pyrolysis

Table VIII. B[a]P concentration in grilled meats, according to their fat content [from *Doremire* et al., 1979]

Meat	Lipids, %	μg of B[a]P/kg	
		mean	extreme values
Turkey	8.3	traces	
Beef	15.0	16.0	13.5–19.2
Beef	19.5	22.8	19.7–26.0
Beef	29.8	30.9	26.1–36.2
Beef	39.1	121.0	90.8–133.2

The meat samples are 1 cm thick and are grilled for 5 min on each side to a 'well-done' state.

being an important contribution to PAH synthesis, the B[a]P level of grilled meats is firstly proportional to their lipid content [*Lijinsky and Shubik,* 1964, 1965; *Lijinsky and Ross,* 1967; *Toth and Blass,* 1973; *Fritz,* 1973; *Doremire* et al., 1979]: in beef meats, an increment of 1% in fat is responsible for a B[a]P enlargement of 1 μg/kg at least (table VIII). (2) To obtain a PAH formation, the lipids must be pyrolyzed in contact with the heat source: fats dripping down from the meat onto hot charcoal or electric resistances generate B[a]P and others PAH. These latter then spread into the atmosphere and are partially deposited on the broiling meat. (3) Consequently, the more fatty the meat is, the more abundant the polymerized products are. The pollution of meat is also inversely proportional to the distance between the heat source and the meat support. (4) To prevent the contamination of grilled meats, an electric resistance and the meat must be opposite to each other – vertically. Thus, the drippings do not fall down onto the heat source and no PAH is formed. With this procedure, grilled sausages only contain 0.5 μg of B[a]P per kg instead of 15.2 μg (30 times more) with the usual manner, sausages being above the heat generator [*Toth and Blass,* 1973]. If such a preventive system cannot be realized, a distance increased between fire and meat and/or strong ventilation are able to reduce the risk of a B[a]P deposit on the broiled product [*Lijinsky and Ross,* 1967; *Toth and Blass,* 1972]. (5) Finally, the heat generator and the combustible category must be considered [*Binneman,* 1979]: every combustible which burns incompletely and with difficulty forms smokes and soots which contain high quantities of PAH and especially B[a]P. That is why fire made of

Table IX. Role of combustible on the B[a]P concentration in grilled meats [from *Toth and Blass,* 1972]

	Grilling over on a fire of					
	wood coal		pine cone		rumpled paper	
	samples	µg/kg	samples	µg/kg	samples	µg/kg
Sausage	3	10.2	1	20.0	1	26.0
Sausage	1	15.2	4	43.5		
Pork loin						
Fatty	3	7.0	1	50.0	1	55.0
Lean	3	4.2	1	140.0	1	70.0
Roast beef	4	0.8	1	18.0	1	25.0

rumpled paper has a strong contaminating effect; if the papers are printed, the B[a]P amounts probably will be enhanced.

In other aspects, coke and wood coal produce little PAH since they have been submitted to treatments which have eliminated the precursors. Resinous woods, inversely, emit much PAH because of their terpenic content. Table IX shows the role of different combustibles on the contamination level of various grilled products; this factor is of high importance in home preparations.

Benzo[a]pyrene in Heated Oils

If the pyrolysis of fatty substances is responsible for B[a]P formation, how does B[a]P evolve in frying, submitted to temperatures lower than those of a pyrolysis phenomenon?

Firstly, an increase of B[a]P in frying oils can occur when the food products are initially rich in this substance; this can partially dissolve in oil during frying: for example, this is probably happening with smoke-cured bacon [*Lintas* et al., 1979].

More generally, a B[a]P decrease is observed in oils heated at temperatures nearly similar to those used in frying: a colza oil heated at 230 °C for 2 h loses two thirds of its B[a]P content [*Fritz,* 1968c]. Heatings of colza or sunflower oils at 285 °C for 10 h are also responsible for a reduction in the B[a]P concentration ranging from 70 to 80% [*Soos,* 1979].

A concrete study made in dough frying shops reveals some B[a]P destruction after use; yet its disappearance is never complete. Its impor-

Table X. Evolution of B[a]P of frying oils in fritter makers [from *Soos,* 1979]

Nature of fat	Duration of heat at 210 °C, h	B[a]P of oil		Acrolein in used oil mg/kg
		before use µg/kg	after use % of loss	
Rapeseed oil	3.5	26.7	68	141
Rapeseed oil	4.0	8.1	49	128
Half rapeseed oil + half lard	15.0	5.7	42	118
Half rapeseed oil + half lard	27.0	5.7	37	80

tance seems directly connected with oxidizability of the medium (table X): with pure rapeseed oil, 1 h of heating is responsible for an average loss of 15%; with a blending of colza oil and lard, the loss is only of about 2%. Moreover, a parallelism is observed between the intensity of both B[a]P destruction and acrolein formation; the two mechanisms are probably dependent on the same oxidative means.

Benzo[a]pyrene in Smoke-Cured Products

Smoke-cured processes are known to enhance the risk for the carcinogenic properties of treated products; some epidemiological investigations have shown a relation between smoke-cured foods and cancer development [*Dungal,* 1961, 1967]. Decision of the authorities of FRG to impose a norm of 1 µg of B[a]P per kg of smoked products has been the motive for numerous analyses to determine the real B[a]P concentrations in these foods [*Toth,* 1971; *Filipovic and Toth,* 1971; *Toth and Blass,* 1972; *Luks and Lenges,* 1973; *Fretheim,* 1976; *Potthast,* 1977, 1978]. According to values reported in table XI, an important percentage of smoked products does not comply with such a requirement. Yet, these values must not overestimate the existence of a potential hazard for the consumer: the B[a]P distribution in smoked products is very selective. It tends to concentrate all upon the surface of the product; its penetration into the matter itself frequently remains small. So this is why the skin of smoked fish contains from 10 to 40 times more B[a]P than the inside flesh does. So it is with the other smoked foods (table XII). This is the reason why the removal of the skin or the superficial layer does constitute a highly favorable technique in the field of healthy quality.

Table XI. B[a]P concentration in commercial smoke-curing products in West Germany [from *Potthast,* 1977]

Food product	Number of Analyses	μg of B[a]P per kg	
		mean	extreme values
Frankfurter sausage	12	0.44	0.18–2.08
Liver sausage	15	0.70	0.15–6.15
Cooked ham			
Black, hot smoking	54	4.07	0.14–56.04
Slight, hot smoking	24	1.67	0.07–12.56
Ham, normal smoking	26	0.29	0.01–1.11
Black ham, cold smoking	22	1.44	0.16–5.60
Raw sausage	87	0.39	0.01–4.56
Ham skin	4	1.87	0.84–3.05
Smoked cheese	3	0.27	0.15–0.38

Table XII. Location of B[a]P in various animal smoke-curing products

Food product	Conditions of smoking	μg of B[a]P/kg		Author
		skin or outside	inside	
Herring	hot, 2 h	35.0	0.94	*Steinig* [1976]
Herring	hot, 2 h	35.5	0.94	*Steinig and Meyer* [1976]
Mackerel	hot, 2 h	25.0	1.2	*Steinig* [1976]
Mackerel	hot, 2 h	24.5	0.65	*Steinig and Meyer* [1976]
Eel	hot, 3 h	61.0	2.8	*Steinig* [1976]
Eel	hot, 3.5 h	67.0	2.95	*Steinig and Meyer* [1976]
Sardine	hot, 2 h	21.0	1.7	*Steinig* [1976]
Whiting		70.0	7.0	*Malanoski* [1968]
Bullhead		0.8	<0.5	*Malanoski* [1968]
Haddock		2.3	traces	*Malanoski* [1968]
Haddock		53.5	4.0	*Malanoski* [1968]
Salmon	cold	3.2	0.45	*Steinig* [1976]
Black Forest ham		0.58	traces	*Toth* [1971]
Bavaria ham		0.67	0.002	*Toth* [1971]
Ham		2.3	0.8	*Malanoski* [1968]
Sausages, meats		5.13	0.23	*Lucisano* et al. [1973]
Cheeses		2.0	0.93	*Lucisano* et al. [1973]

Probably, the penetration rate in the inside of smoked products is greatly facilitated by the lipid content: B[a]P dissolves in this physical phase and thus progresses into the food at a soluble state.

In practice, three main techniques are used for smoke curing: (1) Hot smoking makes use of hot smokes (50–80 °C), directly coming from wood combustion and penetrating in the smoke room without previous cooling. The operation is fast, it lasts 2–5 h according to smoke temperature and to food size. (2) The cold smoking process differs from the former by a previous cooling of smokes before their entrance into the smoke room. The treatment temperatures are between 20 and 40 °C; this entails a longer time for the same result. This procedure was traditionally used for the smoke curing of hams in the hearth. This smoking lasted during several weeks. It brings a very low pollution [*Toth,* 1971; *Potthast,* 1975]. (3) Actually, the 'smoking' can be carried out by means of a liquid smoke into which the foods are immersed. The liquid content gives the product a flavor and a color of the smoke cured.

Usually, the hot procedure pollutes much more than the cold smoking does: herrings respectively contain 2.6 and 0.3 μg of B[a]P per kg [*Lenges* et al., 1976a, 1976b]. This difference is due to the characteristics of smokes used with each technique, hot and cold smokings. The B[a]P is a heavy molecule which easily deposits in solid form. When the smokes are condensed in a state of tars or decanted in soots during cooling, the fraction penetrating in the smoke room is largely impoverished in B[a]P before being in contact with foods [*Lenges,* 1972; *Potthast* et al., 1977]. Therefore, cold smoke curing is a very effective and preventive procedure from a hygiene point of view.

Various other modalities determine the pollution level in the smoked foods: (1) The nature of the wood used for the smoke production is important: resinous woods produce a sooty smoke with high B[a]P concentration; they are to be prohibited [*Potthast,* 1975; *Potthast* et al., 1977]. (2) Burning temperature also takes place: the flavorings and protective components of smokes are more abundant when the combustion temperature is low (about 400 °C). On the contrary, B[a]P emission increases with a temperature increment [*Potthast,* 1975; *Potthast* et al., 1977]. So, it is doubly desirable to lead the burning process to low temperatures. (3) Conditions of smoke emission also give rise to pollution intensity: the longer the distance between the firebox and the smoke room, the poorer the content in B[a]P [*Potthast* et al., 1977]. That is the favorable factor in the cold procedure. (4) In addition to a cooling, a treatment of smoke is a possible way for reducing its harmfulness. For instance, when the smokes are passing through cotton-wool or steel-wool filters, their B[a]P decreases because of particle elimination [*Potthast* et al., 1977]. Smoke washings are also considered in the same way. (5) Finally, the contamination of smoked products originating from the atmosphere will be all the more reduced if the product surface is smaller. In other words, the surface/weight ratio partially causes the B[a]P amount found in smoked foods [*Potthast,* 1975].

In the future, the smoking liquid process might be chosen for its sanitary quality. Some analyses show a nearly total lack of B[a]P: its concentration fluctuates between 0.004 and 1.0 µg per kg [*Engst and Fritz,* 1977]. B[a]P is only found in one of the three smoking products [*Bories* et al., 1978]. It is not detectable in two other smoke liquids [*Lijinsky and Shubik,* 1965]. For their part, two back bacon aroma concentrates contain 2.5 and 1.3 µg of B[a]P per kg [*Engst and Fritz,* 1977].

If these analyses reflect the amounts of almost all the smoke liquids available in industry, their use is a very successful solution from a health point of view, on the condition that drying might not be a cause for pollution.

Conclusion

Beginning with the discovery of fire, some amounts of B[a]P have been produced and released into the atmosphere, with quantities having become especially high in industrialized countries. As a result, the environment is becoming progressively overburdened with numerous PAH which have a carcinogenic property.

Atmospheric photooxidation may be considered as the only natural form of degradation; the pollution observed at the earth's surface proves that more B[a]P is being produced than the atmosphere is capable of degrading. All food vegetal products are polluted to a degree reflecting the amount of B[a]P contained in the atmosphere at the crop site. Consequently, cereals, vegetables and fruits are the main foodstuffs responsible for B[a]P ingestion. These B[a]P concentrations initially present in the crude foodstuffs can be further modified by agronomic and food technologies.

In grains, B[a]P is localized in the outer layers of the pericarp; flour-milling thus removes a major portion of the amount contained in the grain. Bread-making, involving partial oxidation of the remaining B[a]P, exerts a similar action. The oil and fat industry can also reduce a considerable portion of the B[a]P held in crude oils. Blanching and hydrogenation of oils are the most efficient operations. In water assigned for human consumption, deep filtration and dephenolization must be applied in order to obtain an acceptable quality.

At the same time, however, other types of food processing may function to increase the level of pollution. These processes include mainly grilling and roasting at high temperatures and on open fires. In the chemical field, the pyrolysis of fats serves as the main origin of B[a]P formation during heat treatments. This molecule appears most notably with temperatures ranging between 400 and 700 °C; it is generated in such foods as bread crusts, biscuits, and grilled meats.

Finally, every industry using large volumes of air (yeast factory, spray drying) or applying direct smokes (smoke curing, drying by combustion gases) is likely to introduce or enhance the B[a]P concentration on the surface of the treated product.

Studies on food pollution by B[a]P assume particular importance in recognition of the carcinogenic potential of this molecule. On a second level, these studies hold interest as illustrating a case where an economic development, such as industrial and domestic burning and roasting, may have health consequences deserving careful attention.

References

Andelman, J.B.; Suess, M.J.: Polynuclear aromatic hydrocarbons in the water environment. Bull. Wld Hlth Org. *43:* 479–508 (1970).

Andelman, J.B.; Suess, M.J.: The photodecomposition of BP sorbed on calcium carbonate; in Faust, Hunter, Organic compounds in aquatic environment, vol. 1, pp. 439–468 (Dekker, New York 1970).

Beaud, P.; Rollier, H.; Ramuz, A.: Contamination des denrées à l'étalage par la circulation automobile. Trav. chim. alim. hyg. *73:* 196–207 (1982).

Biernoth, G.; Rost, H.E.: The occurrence of polycyclic aromatic hydrocarbons in coconut oil and their removal. Chem. Ind. *45:* 2002–2003 (1967).

Biernoth, G.; Rost, H.E.: Vorkommen polycyclischer aromatischer Kohlenwasserstoffe in Speiseölen und deren Entfernung. Arch. Hyg. Bakt. *152:* 238–250 (1968).

Binnemann, P.H.: Benz[a]pyren in Fleischerzeugnissen. Z. Lebensmitt. Unters. Forsch. *169:* 447–452 (1979).

Bolling, H.: Sostanze cancerogene nei cereali sottoposti ad essiccazione con gas di combustione. Tecnica molitoria. *15:* 137–142 (1964).

Bories, G.: Incidents des façons culinaires sur la contamination des aliments par les hydrocarbures aromatiques polycycliques. Cahier nutr. diet. *17:* 9–16 (1982).

Bories, G.; Tchimbakala, A.; Tchimbakala, E.: Enquête sur la contamination des aliments par le 3,4-benzopyrène. Annls Nutr. Aliment. *32:* 811–818 (1978).

Borneff, J.; Fischer, R.: Kanzerogene Substanz in Wasser und Boden. Untersuchungen an filteraktiver Kohle. Arch. Hyg. Bakt. *145:* 1–11, 334–349 (1961).

Borneff, J.; Kunte, H.: Kanzerogene Substanz in Wasser und Boden. 16. Nachweis von polyzyklischen Aromaten in Wasserproben durch direkte Extraktion. Arch. Hyg. Bakt. *148:* 585–597 (1964).

Borneff, J.; Kunte, H.: Kanzerogene Substanzen in Wasser und Boden. 17. Über die Herkunft und Bewertung der polyzyklischen aromatischen Kohlenwasserstoffe im Wasser. Arch. Hyg. Bakt. *149:* 226–243 (1965).

Borneff, J.; Selenka, F.; Kunte, H.; Maximos, A.: Experimental studies on the formation of polycyclic aromatic hydrocarbons in plant. Environ. Res. *2:* 22–29 (1968).

Bracco, U.: Détermination des hydrocarbures polycycliques aromatiques: technique et application aux huiles de café. Riv. ital. sost. grasse *50:* 166–176 (1973).

D'Arrigo, V.: Idrocarburi policiclici aromatici nelle sostanze grasse. Quad. merceol. *10:* 151–179 (1971).

Davies, W.; Wilmshurst, J.R.: Carcinogens formed in the heating of foodstuffs. Formation of 3,4-benzopyrene from starch at 370–390 °C. Br. J. Cancer *14:* 295–299 (1960).

Depuis, A.: Le problème de l'origine du cancer. Techn. eau. *14:* 25–26 (1960).

Doremire, M.E.; Harmon, G.E.; Pratt, D.E.: 3,4-Benzopyrene in charcoal grilled meats. J. Food Sci. *44:* 622–623 (1979).

Dörr, R.: Die Aufnahme von Alkaloiden und Benzpyren durch intakte Pflanzenwurzeln. Naturwissenschaften *52:* 166 (1965).

Dungal, N.: The special problem of stomach cancer in Iceland. J. Am. med. Ass. *178:* 789–798 (1961).

Dungal, N.; Sigurjonsson, J.: Gastric cancer and diet. A pilot study on dietary habits in two districts differing markedly in respect of mortality from gastric cancer. Br. J. Cancer *21:* 270–276 (1967).

Engst, R.; Fritz, W.: Food hygiene: toxicological evaluation of the occurrence of cancerogenic hydrocarbons in smoked products. Acta alim. pol. *3:* 255–267 (1977).

Fabian, B.: Carcinogenic substances: edible fats and oils. Investigations of margarine, vegetable fat and butter. Arch. Hyg. Bakt. *152:* 231–237 (1968).

Fedorenko, Z.P.: Effect of biochemical treatment of waste-water of a by-product coke plant on their 3,4-benzopyrene content. Gig. Sanit. *29:* 17–19 (1964).

Filipovic, J.; Toth, L.: Polycyclische Kohlenwasserstoffe in geräucherten jugoslawischen Fleischwaren. Fleischwirtschaft *51:* 1323–1325 (1971).

Fretheim, K.: Carcinogenic polycyclic aromatic hydrocarbons in Norwegian smoked meat sausages. J. agric. Fd Chem. *24:* 976–979 (1976).

Fritz, W.: Zur Bildung kanzerogener Kohlenwasserstoffe bei der thermischen Behandlung von Lebensmitteln. 2. Das Rösten von Bohnenkaffee und Kaffee-Ersatzstoffen. Nahrung *12:* 799–804 (1968a).

Fritz, W.: Zur Bildung kanzerogener Kohlenwasserstoffe bei der thermischen Behandlung von Lebensmitteln. 3. Das Backen von Brot und Biskuits. Nahrung *12:* 805–808 (1968b).

Fritz, W.: Zur Bildung kanzerogener Kohlenwasserstoffe bei der thermischen Behandlung von Lebensmitteln. 4. Der Einfluss des Fritierens. Nahrung *12:* 809–811 (1968c).

Fritz, W.: 3,4-Benzpyren und andere Polyaromate in Margarine und Mayonnaise. Nahrung *12:* 495–496 (1968d).

Fritz, W.: Zum Lösungsverhalten der Polyaromate beim Kochen von Kaffee-Ersatzstoffen und Bohnenkaffee. Dt. Lebensm. Rdsch. *65:* 83–85 (1969).

Fritz, W.: Umfang und Quellen der Kontamination unserer Lebensmittel mit krebserzeugenden Kohlenwasserstoffen. Ernährungsforschung *16:* 547–557 (1971).

Fritz, W.: Zur Bildung kanzerogener Kohlenwasserstoffe bei der thermischen Behandlung von Lebensmitteln. 5. Untersuchungen zur Kontamination beim Grillen über Holzkohle. Dt. Lebensm. Rdsch. *69:* 119–122 (1973).

Fritz, W.: Zur Bildung kanzerogener Kohlenwasserstoffe bei der thermischen Behandlung von Lebensmitteln. 6. Untersuchung zur Kontamination bei der direkten Rauchgastrocknung von Getreide. Nahrung *18:* 83–87 (1974).

Fritz, W.: Entstehen bei der Zubereitung von Lebensmitteln krebserzeugende Stoffe? Ernährungsforschung *20:* 49–51 (1975).

Fritz, W.: Untersuchungen über Quellen und Umfang der Kontamination von Lebensmitteln mit polyzyklischen aromatischen Kohlenwasserstoffen sowie Möglichkeiten ihrer Reduzierung; Diss. B, Berlin (1981).

Fritz, W.: Kanzerogene Noxen in der Nahrung unter besonderer Berücksichtigung krebserzeugender Kohlenwasserstoffe. Z. ges. Hyg. Grenzgebiete (in press, 1983).

Fritz, W.; Engst, R.: Kontamination von Lebensmitteln mit krebserzeugenden Kohlenwasserstoffen. Z. ges. Hyg. Grenzgebiete *17:* 271–275 (1971).

Fritz, W.; Uhde, W.J.: Zur Bestimmung von Nitrosaminen in Malz und Bier. Lebensmittelindustrie *29:* 209 (1982).

Gelboin, H.V.; Selkirk, J.; Okuda, T.; Nemoto, N.; Yang, S.K.; Wiebel, F.J.; Whitlock, J.P., Jr.; Rapp, H.J.; Bast, R.C., Jr.: Benzo[a]pyrene metabolism; in Jallow, Kocsis, Snyder, Vainio, Biological reactive intermediates (Plenum Press, New York 1977).

Gräf, W.: Über natürliches Vorkommen und Bedeutung der kanzerogenen polycyclischen aromatischen Kohlenwasserstoffe. Med. Klin. *60:* 561–565 (1965).

Gräf, W.; Diehl, H.: Über den naturbedingten Normalpegel kancerogener polycyclischer Aromate und seine Ursache. Arch. Hyg. Bakt. *150:* 249–259 (1966).

Gräf, W.; Nothhafft, G.: Trinkwasserchlorierung und Benzpyren. Arch. Hyg. Bakt. *147:* 135–146 (1963).

Grigorenko, L.T.; Dikun, P.P.; Kalinina, I.A.; Mironova, A.N.: Effect of commercial hydration and alkali neutralization of edible vegetable oils on their 3,4-benzopyrene content. Trudy Vses Nauchno.-Issl. Inst. Zhirov. *28:* 243–247 (1971).

Grigorenko, L.T.; Mironova, A.N.; Dihun, P.P.: Effect of deodorization of edible vegetable oils on their 3,4-benzopyrene content. Maslozh. Promyshl. *38:* 14–15 (1972).

Grimmer, G.: Entstehen bei der Hitzesterilisierung von Lebensmitteln carcinogene Stoffe? Brot Gebäck *24:* 157–159 (1970).

Grimmer, G.; Duevel, D.: Biosynthetic formation of polycyclic hydrocarbons in the human environment. Z. Naturforsch. *25:* 1171–1175 (1970).

Grimmer, G.; Hildebrandt, A.: Der Gehalt polycyclischer Kohlenwasserstoffe in verschiedenen Gemüsesorten und Salaten. Dt. Lebensm. Rdsch. *61:* 237–239 (1965).

Grimmer, G.; Wilhelm, G.: Der Gehalt polycyclischer Kohlenwasserstoffe in europäischen Hefen. Dt. Lebensm. Rdsch. *65:* 229–231 (1969).

Gunther, F.A.; Buzzetti, F.; Westlake, W.: Residue behavior of polynuclear hydrocarbons on and in oranges. Residue Rev. *17:* 81–104 (1967).

Halaby, G.A.; Fagerson, I.S.: Polycyclic aromatic hydrocarbons in heat-treated foods: pyrolysis of some lipids, beta-carotene and cholesterol. 3rd Int. Conf. Food Sci. Technol., Washington 1970, pp. 820–829.

Handcock, J.L.; Applegate, H.G.; Dodd, J.D.: Polynuclear aromatic hydrocarbons on leaves. Atm. Envir. *4:* 363–370 (1970).

Heffter, A.: Quantitative Bestimmung des 3,4-Benzpyren in Speiseölen. Mitteil. GDCh Fachgruppe Lebensm. Gericht. Chem. *24:* 292–297 (1970).

Howard, J.W.; Fazio, T.: Review of polycyclic aromatic hydrocarbons in foods. J. Ass. off. analyt. Chem. *63:* 1077–1104 (1980).

Howard, J.W.; Fazio, T.; White, R.H.: PAH in solvents used in extraction of edible oils. J. agric. Fd Chem. *16:* 72–76 (1968).

IARC (International Agency for Research on Cancer): Evaluation of carcinogenic risk of the chemical to man. Monogr. IARC 3 (IARC, Lyon 1973).

Ilnitsky, A.P.; Ershova, K.P.; Khesina, A.Y.; Rozhkova, L.G.; Klubkov, V.G.; Korolev, A.A.: Stability of cancerogenic substances in water and the efficacy of methods of its determination. Gig. Sanit. *36:* 8–12 (1971).

Jerina, D.M.; Yagi, H.; Hernandez, O.; Dansette, P.M.; Wood, A.W.; Levin, W.; Chang, R.L.; Wislocki, P.G.; Conney, A.H.: Synthesis and biological activity of potential benzo[a]pyrene metabolites; in Freudenthal, Jones, Carcinogenesis, vol. 1, pp. 91–113 (Raven Press, New York 1976).

Kedzierski, B.: Detection and determination of carcinogenic aromatic polycyclic hydrocarbons. 2. Determination of benzo[a]pyrene in cereals. Prace Inst. Lab. Badawczych. Przem. Spozyw. *25:* 277–285 (1975).

Knorr, M.; Schenk, D.: Zur Frage der Synthese polycyclischer Aromate durch Bakterien. Arch. Hyg. Bakt. *152:* 282–285 (1968).

Kuratsune, M.; Hueper, W.C.: Polycyclic aromatic hydrocarbons in coffee soots. J. natn. Cancer Inst. *20:* 37–51 (1958)

Kuratsune, M.; Hueper, W.C.: Polycyclic aromatic hydrocarbons in roasted coffee. J. natn. Cancer Inst. *24:* 463–469 (1960).

Le Clerc, A.M.; Ramel, P.; Dumain, J.; Fauquembergue, D.: Etude du comportement de quelques matières grasses concrètes au cours d'opérations de friture et de surchauffe contrôlées. Revue fr. Corps Gras. *13:* 175–183 (1966).

Lenges, J.: Le fumage des produits de viande. Rev. ferm. ind. alim. *27:* 53–60 (1972).

Lenges, J.; Luks, D.; Vo Thi, N.B.: Le sodage quantitatif du 3,4-benzopyrène dans les poissons fumés. Rev. ferm. ind. alim. *31:* 20–22 (1976a).

Lenges, J.; Vo Thi, N.B.; Declerck, D.: Influence de la technologie de fumage sur la contamination de poissons fumés en 3,4-benzopyrène. Rev. ferm. ind. alim. *31:* 97–101 (1976b).

Lijinsky, W.; Ross, A.E.: Production of carcinogenic polynuclear hydrocarbons in the cooking of food. Fd Cosmet. Toxicol. *5:* 343–347 (1967).

Lijinsky, W.; Shubik, P.: Benzo[a]pyrene and other polynuclear hydrocarbons in charcoal-broiled meat. Science *145:* 53–55 (1964).

Lijinsky, W.; Shubik, P.: Polynuclear hydrocarbon carcinogens in cooked and smoked foods. Ind. med. Surg. *34:* 152–154 (1965).

Lintas, C.; De Matthaeis, M.C.; Merli, F.: Determination of benzo[a]pyrene in smoked, cooked and toasted food products. Fd Cosmet. Toxicol. *17:* 325–328 (1979).

Lo, M.-T.; Sandi, E.: Polycyclic aromatic hydrocarbons in foods. Residue Rev. *69:* 35–86 (1978).

Lucisano, A.; De Battistis, P.; Marzadori, F.: Ricerca del 3,4-benzopyrene nei prodotti affumicati. Vet. ital. *24:* 232–240 (1973).

Luks, D.; Lenges, J.: Quelques aspects analytiques et pratiques de la contamination de produits de viande fumés par des composants cancérogènes. Rev. ferm. ind. alim. *28:* 111–114 (1973).

McGinnis, E.L.: Determination of four- and five-ring condensed hydrocarbons. 2. Analysis of polynuclear aromatic compounds in *n*-paraffin feed oil for yeast fermentation. J. agric. Fd Chem. *23:* 226–229 (1975).

McGinnis, E.L.; Norris, M.S.: Determination of four- and five-ring condensed hydrocarbons. 1. Analysis of polynuclear aromatic hydrocarbons in yeast produced by growth on both *n*-hydrocarbon and dextrose feeds. J. agric. Fd Chem. *23:* 221–225 (1975).

Malaney, G.W.; Lutin, P.A.; Cibulka, J.J.; Hickerson, L.H.: Resistance of carcinogenic organic compounds to oxidation by activated sludge. J. Water Pollut. Control Fed. *39:* 2020–2029 (1967).

Malanoski, A.J.; Greenfield, E.L.; Barnes, C.J.; Worthington, J.M.; Joe, F.L.: Survey of polycyclic aromatic hydrocarbons in smoked foods. J. Ass. off. agric. Chem. *51:* 114–121 (1968).

Mallet, L.: Pollution par les hydrocarbures des alluvions déposées dans l'estuaire de la Seine à partir de Rouen. Bull. acad. natn. Méd. *146:* 569–575 (1962).

Mallet, L.: Présence des hydrocarbures du type benzo-3,4-pyrène dans les sédiments sous-jacents au lit de la Seine en aval de Paris. Bull. acad. natn. Méd. *149:* 656–666 (1965).

Mallet, L.; Heros, M.: Pollution des terres végétales par les hydrocarbures polybenzéniques du type 3,4-benzopyrène. C.r. Ac. Sci. *254:* 958–960 (1962).

Mallet, L.; Perdriau, L.V.; Perdriau, J.: Pollution par les hydrocarbures polybenzéniques du type benzo-3,4-pyrène de la région occidentale de l'Océan glacial arctique. C.r. Ac. Sci. *256:* 3487–3489 (1963).

Masuda, Y.; Mori, K.; Kuratsume, M.: Polycyclic aromatic hydrocarbons formed by pyrolysis of carbohydrates, amino acids and fatty acids. Gann *58:* 69–74 (1967).

Morimoto, K.; Shibazaki, T.; Inone, T.: Benzo[a]pyrene in dried yeasts. Eisei Shikenjo Hokuku *92:* 63–65 (1974).

Müller, H.: Aufnahme von 3,4-Benzpyren durch Nahrungspflanzen aus künstlich angereicherten Substraten. Z. Pflanzenernähr. Bodenk. *6:* 685–695 (1976).

National Academy of Science: Petroleum in the marine environment (National Academy of Science, Washington 1975).

Poglazova, M.N.; Fedoseeva, G.E.; Khesina, A.Y.; Meisel, H.N.; Shabad, L.M.: About the possibility of benzopyrene destruction by soil microorganisms. Dokl. Akad. Nauk. SSSR *169:* 1174–1177 (1966).

Poglazova, M.N.; Fedoseeva, G.E.; Khesina, A.Y.; Meisel, H.N.; Shabad, L.M.: Metabolism of benzo[a]pyrene by various soil microorganisms and isolated strains. Dokl. Akad. Nauk. SSSR *198:* 348–350 (1972a).

Poglazova, M.N.; Fedoseeva, G.E.; Khesina, A.Y.; Meisel, H.N.; Shabad, L.M.: The microbial degradation of benzo[a]pyrene in waste waters. Dokl. Akad. Nauk. SSSR *204:* 346–348 (1972b).

Potthast, K.: Probleme beim Räuchern von Fleisch und Fleischerzeugnissen. Fleischwirtschaft *55:* 1492, 1494–1496 (1975).

Potthast, K.: Polycyclic aromatic hydrocarbons in smoked meat products. An application of a new method. Acta alim. pol. *3:* 195–201 (1977).

Potthast, K.: Zur Problematik von 3,4-Benzpyren in geräucherten Fleischerzeugnissen. Fleischerei *29:* 69–73 (1978).

Potthast, K.; Eigner, G.; Eichner, R.: Gehalt an polycyclischen Kohlenwasserstoffen in geräucherten Fleischwaren. Ber. Landwirtsch. *55:* 817–822 (1977).

Prokhorova, L.T.; Mironova, A.N.: Occurrence of 3,4-benzopyrene in margarines. Trudy Vses Nauchno.-Issl. Inst. Zhirov. *30:* 36–38 (1973).

Prokhorova, L.T.; Mironova, A.N.; Fal'k, E.Y.: Effect of sunflower oil hydrogenation on the content in 3,4-benzopyrene. Trudy Vses Nauchno.-Issl. Inst. Zhirov. *30:* 33–36 (1973).

Reichert, J.; Kunte, H.; Engelhardt, K.; Borneff, J.: Kanzerogene Substanzen in Wasser und Boden. 27. Weitere Untersuchungen zur Eliminierung kanzerogener, polyzyklischer Aromate aus Abwasser. Arch. Hyg. Bakt. *155:* 18–40 (1971).

Rohrlich, M.; Suckow, P.: Der Einfluss von Trocknung, Lagerung und Verarbeitung auf die 3,4-Benzpyrenmenge in Getreide und Getreidemahlprodukten. Getreide Mehl *20:* 90–93 (1970).

Rohrlich, M.; Suckow, P.: Untersuchungen über 3,4-Benzpyren in Getreide und Versuche zur Verminderung durch die Verarbeitung. Brot Gebäck *25:* 145–147 (1971).

Rohrlich, M.; Suckow, P.: Oxydative Veränderung des 3,4-Benzpyren auf Getreide und in Backwaren. Chem. Mikrob. Technol. Lebensm. *2:* 137–143 (1973).

Santoro, A.; Modica, R.; Paglialunga, S.; Bartosek, I.: Rapid determination of polycyclic aromatic hydrocarbons (PAH) in yeasts grown on *n*-paraffins and molasses. Toxicol. Lett. *3:* 85–93 (1979).

Schamp, N.; Van Wassenhove, F.: Determination of benzo[a]pyrene in bitumen and plants. J. Chromatogr., biomed. Appl. *69:* 421–425 (1972).

Schmeltz, I.; Hoffmann, D.: Carcinogenesis; in Freudenthal, Jones, Polynuclear aromatic hydrocarbons: chemistry, metabolism and carcinogenesis (Raven Press, New York 1976).

Schmidt, F.; Fritz, W.: Studien über Vorkommen und Bildung von polycyclischen aromatischen Kohlenwasserstoffen in Lebensmitteln. G.B.K. Mitteil. *5:* 15–30 (1968).

Shabad, L.M.: On the distribution and the fate of the carcinogenic hydrocarbon benzo[a]pyrene in the soil. Z. Krebsforsch. *70:* 204–210 (1968).

Shabad, L.M.; Cohan, Y.L.: The contents of benzo[a]pyrene in some crops. Arch. Geschwulstforsch. *40:* 237–243 (1972).

Shabad, L.M.; Cohan, Y.L.; Ilnisky, A.P.; Khesina, A.Y.; Shaherbak, N.P.; Smirnov, G.A.: The carcinogenic hydrocarbon benzo[a]pyrene in the soil. J. natn. Cancer Inst. *47:* 1179–1191 (1971).

Siegfried, R.: Einfluss von Müllkompost auf den 3,4-Benzpyren-Gehalt von Möhren und Kopfsalat. Naturwissenschaften *62:* 300 (1975a).

Siegfried, R.: 3,4-Benzpyren in Ölen und Fetten. Naturwissenschaften *62:* 576 (1975b).

Siegfried, R.; Müller, H.: Über die 3,4-Benzpyren-Kontamination von Wurzel- und Blattgemüse aus Böden mit unterschiedlichem 3,4-Benzpyrengehalt. Landwirtsch. Forsch. *31:* 133–140 (1978).

Soos, K.: Gehalt an cancerogenen polyaromatischen Kohlenwasserstoffen in ungarischem Getreide. Z. Lebensmitt. Unters. Forsch. *156:* 344–346 (1974).

Soos, K.: Occurrence of 3,4-benzopyrene in fats and heat-induced changes in its concentration. Acta alim., Budapest *8:* 181–188 (1979).

Soos, K.; Fözy, I.: The content of polyaromatic hydrocarbon carcinogens in various coffee types. Edesipar. *25:* 7–10, 37–40, 65–69 (1974).

Steinig, J.: 3,4-Benzpyren-Gehalt in geräucherten Fischen in Abhängigkeit von Räuchermethode. Z. Lebensmitt. Unters. Forsch. *162:* 235–242 (1976).

Steinig, J.; Meyer, V.: Benzpyren-Gehalte in geräucherten Fischen. Lebensmitt. Wiss. Technol. *9:* 215–217 (1976).

Strobel, R.G.K.: The determination of 3,4-benzopyrene in coffee products. Chim. cafés verts, torr. et dérivés. 6ᵉ coll. ASIC, Bogota 1974, pp. 128–134.

Suess, M.J.: Laboratory experimentation with 3,4-benzopyrene in aqueous systems and the environmental consequences. Z. Bakt. Hyg. Abt. orig. B *155:* 541–546 (1972).

Suess, M.J.: The environmental load and cycle of PAH. Sci. Total envir. *6:* 239–250 (1976).

Swallow, W.: Survey of PAH in selected foods and food additives available in New Zealand. N.Z. J. Sci. *19:* 407–412 (1976).

Takata, T.: From normal paraffin to proteins. Hydrocarb. Process. *48:* 99–103 (1969).

Tilgner, D.J.: Food in carcinogenic environment. Food Manuf. *87:* 47–50 (1970).

Tilgner, D.J.: Cancerogene Kohlenwasserstoffe in Lebensmitteln. Gordian *71:* 2–4 (1971).

Toth, L.: Polycyclische Kohlenwasserstoffe in geräuchertem Schinken und Bauchspeck. Fleischwirtschaft *51:* 1069–1070 (1971).

Toth, L.; Blass, W.: Einfluss der Räuchertechnologie auf den Gehalt von geräucherten Fleischwaren an cancerogenen Kohlenwasserstoffen. 1. Einfluss verschiedener Räucherverfahren. Fleischwirtschaft *52:* 1121–1124 (1972).

Toth, L.; Blaas, W.: Der Gehalt gegrillter Fleischerzeugnisse an cancerogenen Kohlenwasserstoffen. Fleischwirtschaft *53:* 1456–1459 (1973).

Truhaut, R.; Ferrando, R.: The toxicological aspects of single cell proteins used in animal feeding. Proc. Protein-Calorie Advisory Group Symp., Brussels 1976, pp. 38–48.

Vadi, H.; Jernström, B.; Orrenius, S.: Recent studies on benzo[a]pyrene metabolism in rat liver and lung; in Freudenthal, Jones, Carcinogenesis, vol. 1, pp. 45–61 (Raven Press, New York 1976).

Wagner, H.K.; Siddiqi, I.: Die Speicherung von 3,4-Benzfluoranthen in Sommerweizen und Sommerroggen. Z. Pflanzenernähr. Bodenk. *130:* 241–243 (1971).

Woidich, H.; Pfannhauser, W.; Blaicher, G.; Tiefenbacher, K.: Analyse polycyclischer aromatischer Kohlenwasserstoffe in Trink- und Nutzwasser. Mitt. GDCh Fachgruppe Lebensmitt. Ger. Chem. *30:* 141–146 (1976).

J. Adrian, Chaire de Biochimie Industrielle et Agro-Alimentaire, CNAM,
292, rue Saint-Martin, F-75141 Paris Cedex 03 (France)

Wld Rev. Nutr. Diet., vol. 44, pp. 185–211 (Karger, Basel 1984)

Nutritional and Health Implications of Lysine Carnitine Relationship

Mahtab S. Bamji[1]

National Institute of Nutrition, Indian Council of Medical Research, Hyderabad, India

Contents

Introduction

Carnitine (β-hydroxy/γ-butyrobetaine) was discovered towards the beginning of this century from meat extracts by two groups of workers, *Gluwitch and Krimberg* (1905) and *Kutscher* (1905) [1]. Progress in our understanding of this compound has occurred in four distinct phases. Though *Krimberg*, through intuition and reasoning, could make an accurate guess of the chemical nature of carnitine, definite proof of its structure came almost 25 years later through the efforts of some of the best brains in chemistry. *Tomita and Sendju* (1927) separated the two isomers of β-hydroxy, γ-butyrobetaine and demonstrated that the levorotatory isomer was identical with

[1] The author is grateful to Dr. *Jagadeesan* for critical scrutiny of the manuscript. Assistance given by *M. Vijayalaxmi* and *D. Seshadri* in the verification of references is gratefully acknowledged.

the natural carnitine [1]. When acetyl-CoA was discovered in 1930, carnitine (as well as several other quaternary compounds) attracted some attention, but soon the compound was forgotten, until the early 1950s, when *Fraenkel* and co-workers [2, 3] discovered it to be an essential nutrient for the yellow meal worm, and it got the name vitamin Bt. Thus began the third and a vital phase in carnitine research.

Though most organisms and tissues contain carnitine [4, 5], until recently its deficiency symptoms were known to occur only in a few species, such as all the members of the *Tenebrio* family, larva of the yellow fever mosquito *Aedes aegypti,* the beetle *Oryzephilus surinamensis,* a bacterium *Pediococcus soyae* and a carnitine-less mutant of yeast, *Candida bovina* [see 1 for original references]. A few early reports claiming curative effects of carnitine in various types of diseases remain unconfirmed. Recently, however, symptoms of carnitine deficiency have been described in rats and humans. The carnitine requirement of the various organisms that require it for growth differs markedly. Thus, while the *Tenebrio* worms need as much as 0.35 μg/g dry diet, *Torulopsis bovina* needs only 0.2–0.5 μg/100 mg [6].

The fact that carnitine occurs ubiquitously but has vitamin-like properties for only a few organisms whose requirements differ markedly has suggested that it has a vital biological role, and organisms which do not require it synthesise it. The marked variation in the abundance of carnitine in different organisms and in different tissues within an organism has led to the speculation that probably it has more than one biological function [6].

The first clue of the metabolic role of carnitine came from *Bhattacharya* et al. [7] in 1955. They observed that the carnitine analogue, γ-butyrobetaine, inhibited carnitine utilisation by *Tenebrio* larvae. The inhibition was completely reversed by carnitine. Similar observations were made with chick embryo [8]. Concurrently, *Fritz* [9] observed that carnitine could stimulate the oxidation of fatty acids, particularly those having chain lengths greater than C_8, and *Friedman and Fraenkel* [10] discovered an enzyme from pigeon liver, which could reversibly acetylate carnitine by acetyl-CoA.

Carnitine could also stimulate the rate of palmityl-CoA oxidation by mitochondria [11]. The acyl portions of added acyl carnitines, unlike those of acyl-CoA esters, could be readily oxidised by mitochondria [11, 12], suggesting a role of carnitine in the transfer of fatty acyl moieties across the mitochondrial membrane for beta oxidation. Subsequent work showed the participation of mitochondrial carnitine palmitoyl transferases (CPT) in this operation [13–15]. Besides CPT, medium and short chain carnitine acyl

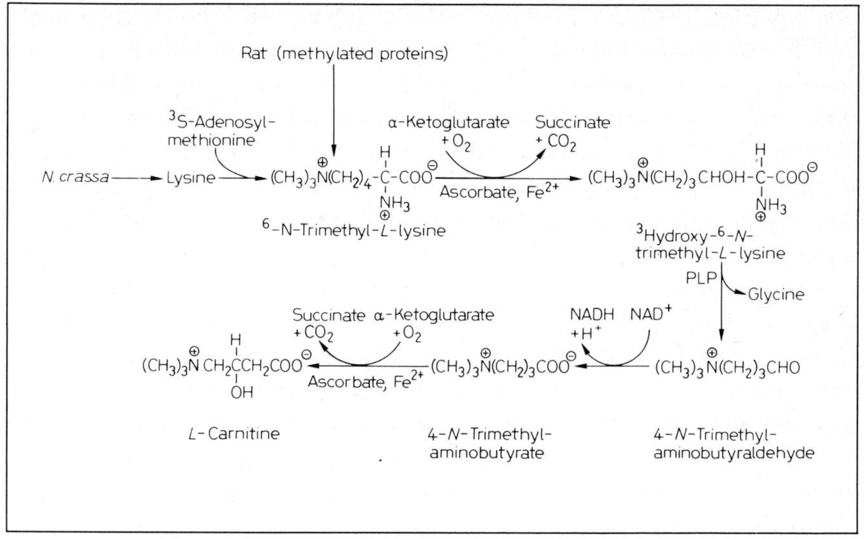

Fig. 1. Pathway of carnitine biosynthesis.

transferases have been described, but their functional significance remains to be elucidated.

More recent studies of *Pande and Parvin* [16, 17] and *Ramsay and Stubbs* [18, 19] show that the acyl carrier role of carnitine requires not only the participation of carnitine acyl transferases, but also of a translocase system for carnitine and its esters.

The fourth phase in the research on carnitine pertains to the discovery of lysine as the precursor of carnitine [20–23]. This has rekindled the interest of nutritionists in carnitine, since lysine is an essential amino acid. If niacin which can be synthesised from tryptophan can be labelled as a vitamin, why not carnitine which is synthesised from lysine?

Biosynthesis of Carnitine

The present understanding of biosynthesis of carnitine in *Neurospora crassa* and rat is described in figure 1. That γ-butyrobetaine (ε-*N*-trimethylamino butyrate, TMAB) is the immediate precursor of carnitine has been known for many years. In 1929, *Linnehweh* observed that TMAB, injected into dogs, produced a rise in urinary carnitine. Many years later, *Lindstedt and Lindstedt* [24] identified and purified an enzyme from rat liver which could hydroxylate TMAB to carnitine. The source of TMAB, however, remained elusive, despite numerous efforts. *Wolf and Berger* [25] injected into rats several labelled intermediates, such as acetate, formate, glycine, glucose, β-hydroxy-4-aminobutyrate, and several essential amino acids including lysine, in the hope of tracing the formation of TMAB, but the label from none of these could be incorporated into carnitine. Similar attempts by other workers also failed. Very slow incorporation of methyl groups of methionine into the methyl groups of carnitine was observed by *Wolf and Berger* [25] and *Bremer* [26]. The incorporation was 15 times higher in choline- and methionine-deficient rats [27]. Thus, it appeared that the methyl groups of carnitine were derived from methionine, but the source of the carbon skeleton remained a mystery. The major breakthrough in this impasse came from the laboratory of *Broquist* who, on the basis of structural similarity, correctly guessed that trimethyl lysine may be a precursor for TMAB [20, 21].

This speculation derived strength from the reports that ε-*N*-trimethyl lysine (TML) residues occur in proteins of plant and animal origin. ε-*N*-di- and trimethyl lysine derivatives have also been found in human urine [28] and ε-*N*-trimethyl lysine and ε-*N*-trimethyl hydroxylysine have been found in the cell walls of diatoms [29]. A mechanism for the cleavage of the glycine moiety of these TMLs would be the key to the biosynthesis of carnitine. Just about that time, *Morley and Stadtman* [30] reported that in *Clostridium sticklandii,* carbon atoms 1 and 2 of lysine are degraded to glycine and the remaining four carbons converted to butyrate.

Initial experiments to test this hypothesis were carried out in the lysine auxotroph of *N. crassa,* strain 33933 [20, 21]. The fungus was grown on a minimal carnitine-less medium, and supplemented with appropriate radioactive test compounds. The biosynthesised carnitine was isolated by ion-exchange column chromatography and its specific activity determined. Suitable isotope dilution experiments using suspected intermediates and precursors showed that radioactivity of *DL*-(6-^{14}C) lysine was incorporated into carnitine without dilution, but radioactivity from *DL*-(1-^{14}C) lysine was not detected in the biosynthesised carnitine. This was the first evidence of a precursor-product relationship between lysine and carnitine. Preliminary data mentioned in the same paper indicated significant isotope dilution of *L*(^{3}HG) lysine incorporation into carnitine, by TML and TMAB, indicating these compounds to be the intermediates in the lysine-carnitine pathway, in *N. crassa*.

The above-mentioned observations coupled with the earlier reports that TMAB could be converted to carnitine in rat [32] and mouse [33], but that γ-aminobutyric acid was not a precursor for TMAB, led to the postulation of the following biosynthetic pathway for carnitine from lysine. Lysine → εNTML → TMAB → carnitine. TMAB would derive its carbon skeleton from C 3, 4, 5 and 6 of lysine, as observed in *Clostridium.* ε-*N*-(^{3}H-methyl) TML could label carnitine very efficiently. ^{3}H-labelled monomethyl and dimethyl lysine were also efficiently incorporated into carnitine, suggesting that *N. crassa* has the mechanism for the stepwise *N*-methylation of lysine, to form TML via monomethyl and dimethyl lysine. Further evidence for this mechanism was obtained by *Rebouch* [41] and *Broquist* [34] using *N. crassa* 38706, a methionine auxotroph. Cell free extracts of this organism could methylate lysine, MML and DML, with *S*-adenosylmethionine as the methyl donor. The enzyme responsible for this methylation has been purified to near homogeneity [35]. *Neurospora* also has a cytochrome *c*-specific protein methylase III which can methylate protein-bound lysine [36]. The early observations in *N. crassa* were extended to rat by *Tanphaichitr and Broquist* [21] and *Cox and Hoppel* [22, 23].

In mammals there is no direct evidence for the methylation of free lysine to TML as in *N. crassa.* The protein methylase III detected by *Paik and Kim* [37] in rat liver suggests that TML may arise from the hydrolysis of methylated proteins. *Labadie* et al. [38] have provided direct evidence for this hypothesis for carnitine biosynthesis in rat. Desialo glycoproteins are known to be rapidly cleared from the blood by the liver, where they are hydrolysed by microsomal proteases. When mono-, di-, or trimethyl-labelled asialofetuin was injected into rats, labelled carnitine was formed only from trimethyl lysine-labelled desialofetuin, but not from mono- and dimethyl lysine-labelled proteins. These results suggest that TML can arise only from the hydrolysis of peptidyl TML, and not from the methylation of free amino acid derivatives.

This inference is in harmony with the observation of *Kakimoto and Akazawa* [28] that urinary excretion of TML did not increase within 2–4 h of oral lysine load. However, more recent studies from the author's laboratory show that in healthy adult human volunteers, plasma carnitine shows significant increase within 3–6 h after the administration of oral lysine [39]. In some subjects, urinary carnitine also showed an increase within 6 h. The phenomenon was specific for lysine and not observed when other amino acids such as tryptophan and threonine were administered. A rapid nonpeptidyl pathway for the formation of carnitine in humans cannot be ruled out. *Strength and Yu* [27] had also observed rapid incorporation of labelled methyl groups of methionine into carnitine in rat, the maximum incorporation being within 3 h of injecting labelled methionine.

The possibility of alternate pathways for generating TML, and probably a species difference in this regard, has been suggested by recent studies of *ElAmin and Means* [40]. These workers administered a casein derivative containing (^{3}H-methyl)-methyl lysine and dimethyl lysine to chickens and analysed the liver and carcass. Almost 60% of the non-protein-bound radioactivity in the liver was found in carnitine, betaine and choline in the ratio 5:3:2. Another 35% was found in protein-bound methionine. From these data, the authors speculated that methyl groups from protein-bound mono- and dimethyl lysine enter the one-carbon pool, by the action of ε-*N*-alkyl lysinase, following protein hydrolysis in the liver. These one carbon fragments are then utilised for the biosynthesis of choline and carnitine via an AdoMet intermediate.

According to *Rebouch* [41], there are some snags in the scheme proposed by *ElAmin and Means* [40]. These are: (a) the abundance of carnitine relative to other methylated cellular metabolites seems rather high, if its synthesis must include incorporation into protein and subsequent hydrolysis; (b) no labelled TML was found in the liver protein hydrolysate; (c) rat liver has the ability to carry out all the transformations proposed in the ElAmin and Means scheme, yet *Labadie* et al. [38] could not detect any conversion of mono- and dimethyl lysine, derived from asialofetuin, to carnitine. It is possible that, unlike the rat, chick can methylate free mono- and dimethyl lysine. Even, then labelled TML should have been detected.

While the measurement of the direct methylation of lysine, mono methyl lysine and dimethyl lysine in chicken liver has not been attempted, such attempts with rat liver and human liver, using the assay condition of *N. crassa,* have failed [41]. It is possible that the assay condition used for *Neurospora* enzyme are not satisfactory for the mammalian activity.

Studies in rat and *N. crassa* suggest that ε-*N*-TML is hydroxylated to β-hydroxy-ε-*N*-TML and then cleaved into γ-*N*-trimethylaminobutyraldehyde and a 2-carbon fragment – a reaction analogous to that of threonine aldolase. The γ-*N*-trimethylaminobutyraldehyde is oxidised to TMAB. Thus, *Hoppel* et al. [42] have detected β-hydroxy-ε-N-TML in the urine of rats injected with methyl-labelled TML. Liver slices could convert β-hydroxy-TML to carnitine. *Hochalter and Henderson* [43] found that rats administered (1-^{14}C) ε-*N*-TML along with hippuric acid excreted radioactive glycine as hippuric acid in the urine. Further evidence that β-hydroxy-ε-*N*-TML and γ-*N*-trimethylaminobutyraldehyde are both intermediates in the lysine-carnitine pathway was obtained through the isotope dilution experiments in *N. crassa* [44]. The most accepted and perhaps the major pathway for the synthesis of carnitine from lysine in *N. crassa* and mammals is described in figure 1.

In vitro experiments with tissue slices suggest that while most tissues can synthesise TMAB only liver and testis can carry out the hydroxylation of TMAB to carnitine [45]. *Carter and Frankel* [46] have examined the relative contributions of different organs to the metabolism of TML in rat. Intravenous injection of tracer dose of (^{3}H-methyl)-TML was given to male rats. At desired time intervals, the animals were killed and total radioactivity in the neutralised perchloric acid extracts measured. A large percentage of the administered label was localised in the kidneys. The kidneys took up 30–50 times more radioactivity than the liver. In nephrectomised animals the incorporation of radioactivity in the liver was markedly lower than in the intact animal. These observations suggested that in the normal animals, not only does the kidney compete for TML, but it contributes significantly to the metabolism of this compound to an intermediate which is later converted to carnitine in the liver.

Chromatographic separation of the intermediates showed that kidneys could synthesise TMAB, but not hydroxylate it to carnitine. Thus, it would appear that in the rat, kidney is the major organ involved in the metabolism of TML to TMAB. In a subsequent study, *Zaspel* et al. [47] examined the interdependence between various tissues for the metabolism of carnitine precursors, using the technique of metabolic vascular perfusion of isolated small intestine, liver, and kidneys. The data suggested that the small intestine absorbs TML efficiently but perhaps plays a negligible role in its metabolism. Kidney absorbs and metabolises TML more readily than the liver. Liver can take up TMAB more rapidly than other tissues and converts it rapidly to carnitine. Thus, it appears that in the rat, kidney plays a major role by supplying to the liver TMAB and the liver completes the synthesis.

Rebouche and Engel [48] have examined the distribution of carnitine biosynthetic enzymes in human tissues obtained at autopsy. Liver and kidney had all the enzymes for carnitine synthesis. Brain also had small amounts of these enzymes, but heart and muscle lacked TMAB hydroxylase. Thus, in humans, kidney would not have to export its TMAB for further conversion to carnitine, but would be expected to act as a major site of carnitine synthesis. In a study in human volunteers, ^{3}H-TML was administered intravenously and labelled metabolites monitored in serum and urine. Nine metabolites were observed. The specific activity of urinary carnitine was greater than serum carnitine. The concentration of labelled carnitine in urine exceeded that of labelled TMAB. In rats the results were opposite [49]. These results point to the importance of kidneys for carnitine synthesis in humans.

Enzymes of the Lysine Carnitine Pathway

S-*Adenosylmethionine:* ε-N-L-*Lysine Methyltransferase. Rebouche and Broquist* [see 34 for the original reference], demonstrated the presence of a time-dependent, protein-dependent activity in cell free extracts of *N. crassa* 33933, which methylated lysine, MML and DML with AdoMet as the methyl donor. The enzyme was purified to near homogeneity [35]. Sedimentation equilibrium and molecular filtration gave a molecular weight of 22,000 for the enzyme protein. No evidence of subunit structure was found.

Protein Methylase III. This enzyme was described by *Paik and Kim* [37, 50] who had earlier described protein methylases I and II. Protein methylase III selectively methylates the ε-amino group of protein-bound lysine. The enzyme has been only partially purified from various vertebrate sources such as calf thymus, calf brain, and chicken embryo. Greater degree of purification has been achieved with protein methylase III from *N. crassa* (3,500-fold) and *S. cerevisiae* (63-fold). While the mammalian enzyme uses histones as the substrate, the *N. crassa* and *S. cerevisiae* enzyme recognises only cytochrome *c* as the substrate.

6-N-*Trimethyl*-L-*Lysine Hydroxylase.* This enzyme catalyses the first reaction in the TML-carnitine pathway (fig. 1). It has been purified 3,700-fold from beef kidney, and requires α-ketoglutarate (αKG) ascorbate and Fe^{2+} as cofactors [51]. Pre-incubation of the enzyme with Fe^{2+} inhibits its activity. This inhibition can be prevented by ascorbate or dithiothreitol, suggesting that ascorbate or dithiothreitol may serve to maintain iron in the ferrous state, thus protecting the hydroxylase from oxidation by ferric iron. While other hydroxylases, such as TMAB hydroxylase, lysine and proline hydroxylase with similar cofactor requirements, occur in microsomes, this enzyme is mitochondrial. Catalase has no effect on TML hydroxylase, though it is known to activate the other hydroxylases, presumably by destroying the H_2O_2 formed in Fe^{2+}-catalysed auto-oxidation of ascorbate. TML hydroxylation is not affected by superoxide dismutase, suggesting that perhaps superoxide is not involved. The K_m for Fe^{2+}, αKG, and TML has been found to be 0.056, 0.22, and 0.13 m*M*, respectively. These values are comparable to that of TMAB hydroxylase, but higher than those for prolyl hydroxylase. It is specific for TML and has no activity on TMAB. Though the enzyme is stable in frozen kidney or frozen mitochondria, the purified enzyme is very unstable.

Serine Transhydroxymethylase. Crystalline serine transhydroxymethylase which acts on several β-hydroxy-α-amino acids such as serine, threonine, allothreonine and a variety of analogs of these acids, was also shown to cleave hydroxy TML. The products of this reaction were shown to be glycine and 4-*N*-trimethylaminobutyraldehyde. The K_m of this enzyme for hydroxy-TML is 3.3 m*M* – a range comparable to that of the other amino acids [51, 52]. The enzyme requires pyridoxal phosphate as a cofactor.

*4-*N*-Trimethylaminobutyraldehyde Dehydrogenase.* This enzyme has been purified to homogeneity from bovine liver [53]. It catalyses the oxidation of trimethylaminobutyraldehyde (TMABA) to TMAB, and requires NAD^+ as a cofactor. While purifying this enzyme, two other aldehyde dehydrogenases were isolated, which did not act on TMABA. The TMABA-specific enzyme is located in the cytosolic fraction. Its K_m for TMABA is 4.2 μ*M*, and has very low activity on propionaldehyde or acetaldehyde. The enzyme is inhibited only 30% by disulfiram at 40 μ*M* concentration. In contrast, the non-specific dehydrogenase of cytosol is inhibited by 83% [52, 53].

TMAB Hydroxylase. Though the last enzyme of the pathway, it was reported almost 15 years ago [24, 33, 54]. As mentioned earlier it uses αKG, Fe^{2+} and ascorbate as cofactors. It has been purified from *Pseudomonas.* Pre-incubation with Fe^{2+} inhibits the enzyme. The explanation given for a similar inhibition of TML hydroxylase may apply to this enzyme as well. The requirement for ascorbate is not absolute. However, ascorbate cannot be replaced by dichlorophenolindophenol and glutathione, as in the case of some other dioxygenases with similar cofactor requirements. Like many other hydroxylases of this kind, TMAB hydroxylase can be stimulated by catalase. Albumin can also stimulate the enzyme. This appears to be a generalised protein effect. Catalase has two types of effects. A generalised protein effect and specific effect due to its catalytic activity. The basis of the catalase effect is not clear, since the bacterial enzyme is not inhibited by hydrogen peroxide. The involvement of the superoxide ions on the enzyme action is not certain.

As mentioned earlier, in the rat, the enzyme is present exclusively in the liver and perhaps testis, but in humans it is present in the kidney as well. On freezing, the liver samples lose their activity. Crude extracts from kidneys of cat, hamster, rabbit and monkey also contain as much or more TMAB hydroxylase activity, but kidneys of other species such as rat, guinea-pig and mouse lack this activity [55, 56].

Examination of human tissues at autopsy suggested that TMAB hydroxylase activity may be age-dependent. In 3 infants the activity was approximately 12% of the normal adult man [41].

Contrary to the mammalian tissues where at least one enzyme, TML hydroxylase is mitochondrial, in *N. crassa* all the enzymes of the lysine-carnitine pathway are in the post-mitochondrial fractions [57].

Tissue Levels and Metabolism of Carnitine

Carnitine content of animal tissues is very much higher than that found in plants and bacteria [1]. Most of the earlier measurements of tissue carnitine were done by the *Tenebrio* assay, which has now been replaced by simpler colorimetric and enzymatic assays [for original references see 58]. A microbiological assay based on the carnitine mutant of the yeast *Torulopsis bovina* has been described [59] but the mutant is unstable and reverts to the wild type easily [*Prabhakar and Polasa,* personal communication]. A gas chromatographic method has also been described [60]. It tends to give higher values than the enzymatic assay [58]. Due to methodological differences of extraction and estimation the values described from different laboratories for the same tissue differ. Since, till recently, only *D,L*-carnitine standards were available, many workers report the values as *D,L*-carnitine, which are twice as high as the actual value of the biologically active form-*L*-carnitine. Tissues such as heart and muscle which derive most of the energy from fat, have the highest concentration of carnitine, whereas brain has the lowest content [61].

Isotope dilution data favour a two-compartment model for carnitine turnover and metabolism in rat [62, 64]. The synthesis of carnitine in the rat has been calculated to be 2 μmol/100 g body weight/day [63, 64]. Under normal conditions very little carnitine is metabolised. Intact carnitine is excreted in the urine. In some physiological states such as cold stress, starvation diabetes, and pregnancy, decarboxylation of carnitine to 5-methylcholine has been reported, but this observation needs confirmation [65].

In rat plasma, carnitine levels are controlled by sex hormones. While androgens raise the level, oestrogens tend to lower it. Thus, adult males tend to have higher levels than adult females [66]. *Mitchell* [67] has reviewed the factors which influence carnitine levels in human body fluids. Serum carnitine is mostly present as free carnitine and short chain acyl carnitine [68].

Hoppel et al. [69] have examined changes in plasma carnitine and acyl carnitines (acid-soluble short chain, and acid-insoluble, long chain) in various metabolic studies. They suggest that to understand carnitine's role, it is essential to measure all these fractions. Plasma total carnitine and carnitine were found to decrease when carnitine intake was reduced in humans [69]. Fasting raised plasma total carnitine, due to increase in acyl carnitines and a delayed fall in carnitine. States of accelerated ketogenesis such as diabetic ketosis and ketoacidosis also reduced carnitine but raised acyl carnitine. Somatostatin infusions had similar effects due to an abrupt reduction in insulin. A patient with elevated levels of long chain acyl carnitine levels was found to suffer from a deficiency of CPT activity in the muscle.

Urinary excretion of carnitine tends to be lower in women than in men. Prolonged fasting tends to raise urinary carnitine in humans as it does in rats, but shorter duration of fasting may have the opposite effect. Strenuous exercise also tends to increase urinary carnitine, but such an increase may not be observed in a trained athlete. Information on concurrent changes in urinary and muscle carnitine in relation to exercise is not available, either in humans or in rats, but data in rats suggest that routine exercise does not increase the carnitine requirement of adequately fed animals [70].

Carnitine Deficiency and Its Effects

From the above discussion one can speculate that carnitine deficiency may arise in dietary deficiency of either of the precursor amino acids (lysine and methionine) or any of the cofactors (iron, ascorbic acid, pyridoxine and niacin) required by the enzymes of the lysine-carnitine pathway (fig. 1).

Liver and kidney dysfunction could also impair carnitine synthesis. Apart from defective synthesis other factors such as increased metabolic losses due to catabolism, impaired kidney tubular resorption, defective transport machinery for transporting carnitine from the tissues where it is synthesised (liver, kidney) to the tissues where it is maximally utilised (muscle, heart) and defective uptake by the tissues may also lead to carnitine deficiency syndrome. A high fat diet would increase carnitine requirement. While carnitine deficiency due to metabolic or transport factors is still speculative, carnitine deficiency due to deficiency of some of the essential nutrients has been demonstrated in experimental animals, and teleologically inferred in man. Case reports of lipid myopathies due to genetic defects in carnitine synthesis, and transport and carnitine deficiency due to liver and kidney diseases in humans have appeared.

Carnitine Status in Malnutrition. Tissue carnitine deficiency has been shown to occur in rats fed on cereal diets which are known to be deficient in essential amino acids, particularly lysine [21, 71–73]. When male weanling rats were fed wheat gluten [21, 81] or whole wheat [72] diets limiting in lysine and threonine, carnitine content of tissues such as skeletal muscle [21, 71, 72], heart, and plasma were lower, but liver carnitine levels tended to be higher compared to the casein diet-fed [72] or laboratory chow-fed rats [21, 74]. Skeletal muscle and kidney levels of carnitine were also found to reduce on a rice diet [73]. Supplementation of these cereal-protein-based diets with lysine and threonine or carnitine produced improvement in skeletal muscle, heart and kidney carnitine. Plasma carnitine improved, when the wheat gluten diet was supplemented with 0.8% lysine and threonine [71] but tended to reduce further when wheat diet was supplemented with a mixture of 0.2% lysine and 0.2% threonine [72]. These apparently contradictory findings with regard to plasma carnitine can be rationalised, if one takes into account the factor of growth. For the same intake of food, the amino acid supplemented rats grow more rapidly, and hence perhaps require more carnitine. A higher supplement of 0.8% lysine may be able to fulfil the need for growth and additional carnitine synthesis, whereas with a lower level of lysine supplement, tissues would abstract carnitine from the plasma.

That a fall in tissue carnitine levels may have a physiological significance is apparent by the fact that in the above-described experiments [21, 71–73], cereal protein diets produced significant accumulation of lipids in tissues such as muscle, heart, plasma and even liver. Supplementation with either carnitine or the limiting amino acids, lysine and threonine, reduced the lipid load of the tissues. In the experiment with whole wheat diet [72], the rise in tissue lipids was associated with impaired in vitro oxidation of palmitate by the heart homogenates, suggesting impaired oxidation of fat as the underlying cause for the rise in tissue lipids.

While these observations follow an expected trend, there are also some intriguing findings. For instance, the lipid concentration of the liver was higher on cereal based diets, despite slightly elevated carnitine levels. Assuming that the rise in liver lipids was due to inadequate synthesis of lipoproteins for mobilising liver lipids, and increase in liver carnitine was also due to defective mobilisation, it is not clear how the administration of carnitine in the diet could reduce the lipid load of the liver. Likewise, in the experiments of *Khan and Bamji* [72], the carnitine content of heart did not fall significantly on wheat diet, yet palmitate oxidation was impaired and lipid levels rose. Supplementation of the wheat diet with the limiting amino acids, or carnitine produced only insignificant increase in heart carnitine, but a significant improvement in palmitate oxidation and fall in lipid levels. It is possible that the two pools of carnitine (indicated by the turnover studies) behave differently to dietary manipulations. The fatty acid oxidation in the heart homogenates of wheat-fed rats could not be fully corrected by exogenous carnitine, suggesting that carnitine deficiency may affect the functional integrity of the fatty acid oxidation system in more than one way.

In a recent study, the effects of maternal dietary lysine deficiency on tissue carnitine levels of mother and fetus were examined [74]. No significant reduction in carnitine levels of maternal plasma and liver or fetal plasma and liver were observed. On the contrary, the levels tended to be higher in the lysine-deficient group. These ambiguous results may again be due to the difference in the growth of the animals in the two groups. Data on skeletal muscle carnitine levels are not reported.

In growing animals nutritional factors that limit carnitine biosynthesis also limit growth and thereby reduce carnitine requirement. In lysine deficiency, the catabolism of lysine to saccharopine is reduced [75]. This may make more lysine available for carnitine synthesis. Additionally, kidney has an efficient mechanism for salvaging TML from tissues. Less than 0.2% lysine is converted to carnitine [76]. In view of these considerations, demonstration of carnitine deficiency in rats fed on cereal-protein diets which are only mildly deficient in lysine is surprising.

Reports on the effects of dietary methionine deficiency on carnitine nutriture are conflicting. *Khairallah and Wolf* [77] found that rats fed a low-protein diet limiting in methionine grew poorly and developed fatty livers. Supplementation with carnitine improved growth and reduced the fat content of the liver. However, *Tsai* et al. [63] calculated that less than 5% of methionine requirement of rats is needed for daily carnitine synthesis of 1.5 μmol/100 g body weight, and hence an effect of carnitine on growth in methionine-deficient rats is unlikely.

In humans, plasma carnitine levels have been observed to decline in severe forms of protein-calorie malnutrition [78–80] and malnutrition in children and adults due to schistosomiasis infection [81]. However, apparently healthy adult Indian men of low income groups, subsisting on cereal diets, had similar levels of plasma carnitine as men of high income groups, despite significantly lower lysine and carnitine intake by the former group [80]. This would imply that the cereal-based diets of low income group Indians provide enough lysine for carnitine synthesis. The low fat content of the low income group diets may have reduced the requirement for carnitine.

Quantity and quality of dietary fat have been reported to modify total, free and acyl carnitine levels in plasma. *Khan-Siddiqui and Bamji* [80] observed that daily supplement of 25 g butter fat to low income group Indians whose habitual diets were very low in fat, produced a small but significant fall in plasma total and free carnitine, but a slight rise in acyl carnitine. The latter suggests that carnitine was being utilised for fat metabolism. *Konig* et al. [82] have also reported a fall in plasma total carnitine levels after oral and intravenous administration of fats containing long-chain fatty acids to humans. In rats, high fat diet containing long-chain fatty acids reduced free as well as total carnitine, but medium-chain fatty acids produced a fall in free carnitine and a rise in acyl carnitine [83].

A weak inverse correlation has been observed between body weight/height^2 ratio (anthropometric index) and plasma carnitine levels in apparently healthy men [80]. From these results, it appears that plasma carnitine levels may be regulated by factors that determine its availability (dietary carnitine, or synthesis) and utilisation (body weight, dietary fat) [80]. Since individuals who consume carnitine- or lysine-deficient diets also tend to consume less fat and are small in stature, carnitine deficiency would be a relatively less common event, and not seen in milder forms of malnutrition.

In a recent survey of the Thai population [84], plasma as well as urinary carnitine levels were found to be higher in adult men from Bangkok, compared to those from Ubol, a rural province in northeast Thailand. Though both the populations subsisted on rice as the staple, the Ubol population was more undernourished, as judged by lower levels of urinary creatinine, serum albumin, and haematocrit. These observations in the Thai population are at some divergence to the observations reported on adult Indian men, where marginal malnutrition tended to raise the plasma carnitine levels [80]. Information on the fat intake in the rural and urban Thai population would help to understand the basis of the different trends.

The significance of the fall in plasma carnitine concentration in severe protein-calorie malnutrition (PCM) in humans is not clear. While lipid myopathy has not been reported in PCM, fatty changes in the liver are known to occur in PCM. According to one report, in kwashiorkor, the heart becomes flabby and vacuolated [85]. This may be due to lipid accumulation besides oedema. Advanced cases of schistosomiasis show a rise in the level of free fatty acids in the serum, suggesting disturbances in lipid metabolism.

Reduced availability of the precursor amino acids, lysine and methionine may be one of the many factors responsible for the fall in plasma and tissue carnitine levels in PCM. Deficiency of other nutrient cofactors such as ascorbic acid, iron, pyridoxine and niacin may also contribute, since they invariably coexist in PCM. Ascorbic acid deficiency in guinea pigs has been found to diminish muscle carnitine levels and increase triglyceride levels [86]. *Nelson* et al. [87] have examined the in vivo conversion of carnitine precursors, TML and TMAB to carnitine, in normal and scorbutic guinea pigs. The conversion of ^{14}C-TML to TMAB in the kidneys was 8–10 times greater in the control animals compared to the scorbutic animals. On the other hand, the hydroxylation of TMAB, which occurred only in the liver, was not affected by ascorbic acid deficiency. Thus, it would appear that ascorbic acid deficiency affects TML hydroxylase to a greater extent than the hydroxylation of TMAB.

Dunn et al. [88] examined the effect of pyridoxal phosphate (PLP) deficiency on carnitine synthesis from lysine, in perfused rat liver, by using PLP antagonist *l*-amino-*D*-proline. The total production of TMAB from protein-bound TML was depressed by 60–80% in the presence of the inhibitor. The decreased synthesis of carnitine was accompanied by an accumulation of 3-hydroxy-6-*N*-TML, the precursor of TMAB in the carnitine biosynthetic pathway. The effects of the inhibitor could be completely reversed by the inclusion of pyridoxine in the perfusion medium. As mentioned earlier, pyridoxal phosphate is a cofactor for the enzyme serine transhydroxymethylase, which catalyses the conversion of TML to trimethyl aminobutyraldehyde.

According to an earlier study, choline deficiency leads to carnitine depletion, presumably through depletion of methyl groups [89]. The observation needs to be confirmed.

Carnitine Status of Mother and Fetus. Carnitine levels of pregnant women tend to be lower than those of the non-pregnant women, particularly in the last trimester [90, 91]. Cord blood levels are higher than the maternal blood suggesting an active process for transplacental transport of carnitine. Carnitine level of milk increases during the first week postpartum. After 1 month, the values tend to decline. Carnitine nutrition would be of considerable importance to an infant, particularly new-born who is suddenly exposed to a high fat maternal milk diet after being used to deriving its nourishment in utero, primarily from maternal glucose [92]. There is a direct correlation between maternal blood and cord blood carnitine at birth [93]. Thus, the adequate carnitine status of the mother is important for the new-born infant's well-being. Plasma levels of carnitine rapidly decrease in premature new-borns during the first 3 days after birth if no exogenous carnitine is given [93]. Some milk formulas, which are based on soy protein, tend to be low in carnitine. One can expect carnitine deficiency in such infants [94]. *Novak* et al. have observed lower levels of plasma carnitine in infants receiving soy-protein-based formulas than those receiving breast milk or cow's milk. The physiological significance of this is not clear. However, the plasma concentration of 3-hydroxybutyrate has been found to be significantly lower in infants fed on soy-based formulas [96]. This is of significance since carnitine is essential for hepatic ketogenesis to occur. The effect of maternal malnutrition on milk carnitine levels and fetal carnitine status needs to be investigated. Absorption of carnitine is believed to be better from maternal milk than formula milk [97].

Carnitine Deficiency in Liver Diseases. As discussed earlier, liver is the major site for carnitine synthesis in man and animals. In certain species, such as rat, guinea-pigs and mouse the last enzyme of the carnitine biosynthetic pathway, namely trimethyl aminobutyrate hydroxylase, is present only in the liver. Information on carnitine nutriture in liver diseases is very scanty and contradictory. *Rudman* et al. [98, 99] examined the carnitine status of 255 hospital patients, and found low levels of plasma carnitine in 30% of the patients suffering from liver cirrhosis. Cirrhotic patients also exhibited anorexia and were generally malnourished. To differentiate between the roles of exogenous (dietary) and endogenous (biosynthetic) factors in the causation of hypocarnitinaemia in cirrhotics, an excess supply of precursor amino acids was given to the patients and controls. In the patients, plasma carnitine levels failed to normalise whereas the controls maintained the levels. From these results the authors conclude that the hepatocellular disease blocks the pathway for biosynthesis of carnitine. Postmortem examination of patients who died of cirrhosis revealed low levels of liver carnitine, suggesting that impaired mobilisation from the liver may not be the reason for carnitine deficiency in cirrhotics. Muscle atrophy, fatty liver and neurological disturbances of cirrhotic patients may be aetiologically related to carnitine deficiency [98, 99].

Hoppel et al. [69] have failed to confirm the findings of *Rudman* et al. [98, 99]. On the contrary, they found significant elevation in total and acyl carnitine levels in the plasma of a majority of cirrhotics, compared to the controls. Free carnitine levels were also elevated in a few patients, but were within the normal range in the others [69]. The reasons for such divergent findings are not clear.

Carnitine Deficiency in Kidney Diseases. Kidney can influence carnitine nutriture in two ways – synthesis and excretion. Several of the patients of renal insufficiency have been reported to have higher levels of plasma carnitine, compared to controls. However, patients undergoing haemodialysis develop hypocarnitinaemia as suggested by low levels of plasma and muscle carnitine [100–103]. The effect is transient (in some patients) and values return to normal or above-normal levels, approximately 6 h after dialysis, whereas in others the low levels persist [102]. Administration of *D,L*-carnitine orally at the end of the dialysis or its addition to the dialysate helps to maintain blood levels [103].

Patients undergoing haemodialysis show elevated levels of plasma triglycerides. Administration of *D,L*-carnitine orally helps to normalise triglyceride levels without producing any adverse effects [104–106]. Treatment with *D,L*-carnitine or thiadenol, though less effective than clofibrate, has been found to be safer and more desirable in chronic uraemia [107]. Symptoms of myasthenia have been observed in some patients who received intravenous injections of very high doses (2 g) of carnitine [108].

Bohmer et al. [101] suggest that the syndrome of cardiomyopathy and cardiac failure observed in some patients undergoing dialysis may be due to carnitine deficiency. Since muscle carnitine levels are also reduced in patients undergoing haemodialysis, the status of patients undergoing haemodialysis should be monitored, and appropriate corrective therapy given.

Lipid Myopathies. In 1963, *Engel and Angelini* reported a case of muscle dystrophy, associated with lipid accumulation and impaired ability to oxidise long chain fatty acids. The carnitine concentration of the muscle was very low in these patients. In vitro addition of carnitine restored the fatty acid oxidising capacity. Since then over 28 such cases have been described [for original references, see 108, 109]. In all the cases, there was weakness and lipid accumulation in the muscle, particularly in the type I fibres, accompanied by low carnitine concentration in the muscle. However, only some patients showed low levels of carnitine in liver and plasma, suggesting that the patients differed with respect to the type of biochemical defect. *Broquist and Borum* [109] have summarised the individual case histories of the 28 cases reported in the literature.

Three types of biochemical defects are believed to produce carnitine deficiency and concomitant lipid myopathy. These are: (1) defective synthesis in the liver (low carnitine levels in muscle, liver and plasma, systemic deficiency); (2) defective uptake by the muscle (low levels in muscle but normal levels in plasma and liver); (3) defective release from the liver (low levels in muscle and plasma, systemic deficiency) but normal or higher levels in liver. These defects are believed to be genetic. Some of the patients responded to treatment with prednisone and some to carnitine.

Relatively low levels of carnitine have also been observed in the muscle of patients suffering from other types of myopathies, such as Duchenne dystrophy and Becker dystrophy [109].

Rebouch and Engel [110] have examined the biosynthesis of carnitine from (^{3}H-methyl) TML in patients of systemic carnitine deficiency. Their results suggest that carnitine synthesis is not affected in these patients and that the metabolic defect may lie outside the biosynthetic pathway. They feel that abnormal renal absorption may be one of the factors responsible for systemic carnitine deficiency.

Effects of Carnitine Deficiency on Heart. Fatty degeneration of the heart, along with a fall in carnitine concentration and impaired fatty acid oxidation, has been observed in guinea-pigs infected with diphtheria toxin [111]. In vitro studies show that diphtheria toxin inhibits the transport of carnitine into an established cell line from human heart, by inhibiting the synthesis of carriers. Addition of prednisolone to the medium, along with the toxin, opposed this effect of the toxin [112].

Relatively large amounts of carnitine have been reported to be lost from ischaemic myocardium [for original reference see 113]. Administration of carnitine is believed to have a beneficial effect [114]. Myocardial carnitine deficiency has been observed in chronic heart failure. According to *Suzuki* et al. [114], the beneficial effect of *L*-carnitine on ischaemic heart may be due to restoration of energy metabolism of ischaemic myocardium and preventing ventricular arrhythmias.

Other Functions of Carnitine

In addition to its role in the translocation of long chain acyl residues, across the inner membrane of mitochondria, carnitine is also believed to have other roles – perhaps indirectly connected with the carnitine-acyl carnitine antiport system.

Branched Chain Ketoacid Metabolism. Branched chain keto acids are derived by transamination of branched chain amino acids such as leucine, isoleucine and valine by the enzymes branched chain amino acid transaminase. Carnitine has been found to stimulate branched chain keto acid oxidation by removing the product acyl-CoA inhibition of branched chain fatty acid dehydrogenase (located on the inner surface of the inner mitochondrial membrane) by releasing CoA [115]. In protein calorie malnutrition and starvation, muscle proteins are utilised for deriving energy. The impact of carnitine deficiency in PCM, on this process, merits investigation.

Male Reproduction. Carnitine is believed to have more than one functional role in male reproduction. The epididymidis of several species of animals and humans has been found to contain high concentrations of carnitine [116]. It is present mostly in the luminal fluid, and attains the highest concentrations in the cauda segment. Such high concentrations are achieved by extraction and accumulation from the plasma, rather than synthesis [116]. The epididymidis derives a considerable amount of energy from lipids – perhaps glycerylphosphorylcholine which accumulates in the epididymidis. Activities of carnitine palmitoyl-transferase as well as carnitine acetyltransferase, in the epididymidis, are under androgen control.

Carnitine appears to play an important role, even in sperm metabolism [117]. The intracellular concentration of carnitine and acetylcarnitine in mature spermatozoa is very high. Surprisingly long chain acylcarnitine is not detectable. Spermatozoa depend upon exogenous fatty acids and endogenous phospholipids for energy and carnitine may help in this process. In the epididymal spermatozoa, carnitine may also depress respiration by altering the acetyl-CoA:CoA equilibrium. This would restrict the activity of the tricarboxylic acid cycle, and depress the metabolic activity of epididymal sperms. The availability of glycolytic substrates is very low in the epididymidis.

In the highly motile ejaculated sperms, acetyl carnitine would act as a ready substrate for energy. Pyruvate plays a key role in maintaining the supply of acetylcarnitine.

The relationship between carnitine and the sperm-specific LDH-X is not clear. LDH-X, unlike other LDH isozymes, can act on longer chain keto acids as well. This may enlarge the scope of available energy-yielding substrates for the sperms. Carnitine may facilitate the metabolism of these acids by their translocation into the mitochondria as well as by removing the inhibition of α-keto acid dehydrogenases in the mitochondria, by acyl-CoA, and release CoA for further metabolism. Such a role for carnitine in the metabolism of branched chain keto acids was discussed earlier. Carnitine may also help to transport, out of the mitochondria, acetyl moieties for the synthesis of acetyl choline – essential for sperm motility.

A direct correlation between the carnitine content of the sperms and fertility has been observed in bulls. The effect of carnitine deficiency, due to causes discussed earlier, on male reproduction needs to be investigated.

Summary

Trimethyl lysine (TML) is a precursor for carnitine in *Neurospora crassa* and mammals. Cofactor requirement for iron, ascorbic acid and pyridoxal phosphate is indicated for the various enzymatic reactions of the TML-carnitine pathway. Experimental studies in animals suggest that deficiencies of lysine, ascorbic acid or pyridoxine may lead to a fall in plasma and/or tissue carnitine levels. A rise in tissue lipids due to lysine deficiency in rats can be corrected by giving carnitine orally. Severe forms of protein calorie malnutrition in humans lead to a fall in plasma carnitine levels. Sex hormones, body size and dietary lipids are among the other factors that regulate plasma carnitine levels.

In rats, TML has to be derived from the breakdown of methylated proteins, since free lysine cannot be methylated. In humans, however, oral administration of lysine raises plasma and urinary carnitine within 3–6 h, indicating the possibility of a non-peptidyl pathway for generating TML. Malnutrition abolishes such a rise. Liver is the major site for the synthesis of carnitine in rat, since the terminal hydroxylase (trimethyl aminobutyrate hydroxylase) is absent from most tissues. In several other species, including humans, kidney also contains this enzyme and hence can synthesise carnitine. Carnitine deficiency in humans can be expected in diseases of the liver and kidney, but the data are equivocal. Case reports of lipid myopathies due to genetic defects in carnitine synthesis or utilisation are available. Carnitine appears to have more than one functional role in male reproduction.

References

1 Friedman, S.; Fraenkel, G.S.: Carnitine; in Sebrell, Harris, The vitamins, vol. 5, pp. 329–355 (Academic Press, New York 1972).

2 Fraenkel, G.: B_T, a new vitamin of the B-group and its relation to the folic acid group and other anti-anaemia factors. Nature, Lond. *161:* 981–983 (1948).

3 Carter, H.E.; Bhattacharyya, P.K.; Weidman, K.R.; Fraenkel, G.: Chemical studies on vitamin B_T. Isolation and characterization as carnitine. Archs Biochem. Biophys. *38:* 405–416 (1952).

4 Fraenkel, G.: Effect and distribution of vitamin B_T. Archs Biochem. Biophys. *34:* 457–467 (1951).

5 Fraenkel, G.: The distribution of vitamin B_T (carnitine) throughout the animal kingdom. Archs Biochem. Biophys. *50:* 486–495 (1954).

6 Fraenkel, G.: The proposed vitamin role of carnitine; in Fraenkel, McGarry, Carnitine biosynthesis, metabolism and functions, pp. 1–6 (Academic Press, New York 1980).

7 Bhattacharyya, P.K.; Friedman, S.; Fraenkel, G.: The effect of some derivatives and structural analogs of carnitine on the nutrition of *Tenebrio molitor.* Archs Biochem. Biophys. *54:* 424–431 (1955).

8 Ito, T.; Fraenkel, G.: Anti-carnitine effect of γ-butyrobetaine on the development of the chick embryo. Fed. Proc. *15:* 558 (1956).

9 Fritz, I.B.: Factors influencing the rate of long-chain fatty acid oxidation and synthesis in mammalian systems. Physiol. Rev. *41:* 52–129 (1961).

10 Friedman, S.; Fraenkel, G.: Reversible enzymatic acetylation of carnitine. Archs Biochem. Biophys. *59:* 491–501 (1955).

11 Fritz, I.B.; Yue, K.T.N.: Long-chain carnitine acyltransferase and the role of acylcarnitine derivatives in the catalytic increase of fatty acid oxidation induced by carnitine. J. Lipid Res. *4:* 279–288 (1963).

12 Bremer, J.: Carnitine in intermediary metabolism. J. biol. Chem. *237:* 3628–3632 (1962).

13 Chase, J.F.A.; Pearson, D.J.; Tubbs, P.K.: The preparation of crystalline carnitine acetyltransferase. Biochim. biophys. Acta *96:* 162–165 (1965).

14 Norum, K.R.: Palmityl-CoA: carnitine palmityl transferase purification from calf-liver mitochondria and some properties of the enzyme. Biochim. biophys. Acta *89:* 95–108 (1964).

15 Norum, R.K.; Bremer, J.: The localization of acyl co-enzyme A-carnitine acyltransferases in rat liver cells. J. biol. Chem. *242:* 407–411 (1967).

16 Pande, S.V.; Parvin, R.: Characterization of carnitine acylcarnitine translocase system of heart mitochondria. J. biol. Chem. *251:* 6683–6691 (1976).

17 Pande, S.V.: A mitochondrial carnitine acylcarnitine translocase system. Proc. natn. Acad. Sci. USA *72:* 883–887 (1975).

18 Ramsay, R.R.; Tubbs, P.K.: The mechanism of fatty acid uptake by heart mitochondria: an acyl carnitine-carnitine exchange. FEBS Lett. *54:* 21–25 (1975).

19 Ramsay, R.R.; Tubbs, P.K.: The effects of temperature and some inhibitors on the carnitine exchange system of heart mitochondria. Eur. J. Biochem. *69:* 299–303 (1976).

20 Horne, D.W.; Tanphaichitr, V.; Broquist, H.P.: Role of lysine in carnitine biosynthesis in *Neurospora crassa.* J. biol. Chem. *246:* 4373–4375 (1971).

21 Tanphaichitr, V.; Broquist, H.P.: Lysine deficiency in the rat: concomitant impairment in carnitine biosynthesis. J. Nutr. *103:* 80–87 (1973).

22 Cox, R.A.; Hoppel, C.L.: Biosynthesis of carnitine and 4-*N*-trimethyl aminobutyrate from lysine. Biochem. J. *136:* 1075–1082 (1973).

23 Cox, R.A.; Hoppel, C.L.: Biosynthesis of carnitine and 4-*N*-trimethyl aminobutyrate from 6-*N*-trimethyl lysine. Biochem. J. *136:* 1083–1090 (1973).

24 Lindstedt, G.; Lindstedt, S.: Cofactor requirements of γ-butyrobetaine hydroxylase from rat liver. J. biol. Chem. *245:* 4178–4186 (1970).

25 Wolf, G.; Berger, C.R.A.: Studies on the biosynthesis and turnover of carnitine. Archs Biochem. Biophys. *92:* 360–365 (1961).

26 Bremer, J.: Biosynthesis of carnitine in vivo. Biochim. biophys. Acta *48:* 622–624 (1961).

27 Strength, D.R.; Yu, S.Y.: Origin of methyl group of carnitine (Abstract). Fed. Proc. *21:* 1 (1962).

28 Kakimoto, Y.; Akazawa, S.: Isolation and identification of N^G,N^G- & N^G,N^{1G}-dimethyl arginine, *N*-mono, di- and trimethyl lysine, and glucosyl galactosyl hydroxylysine from human urine. J. biol. Chem. *245:* 5751–5758 (1970).

29 Nakamima, T.; Volcani, B.E.: ε-*N*-trimethyl-*L*-8-hydroxylysine phosphate and its non-phosphorylated compound in diatom cell walls. Biochem. biophys. Res. Commun. *39:* 28–33 (1970).

30 Morely, C.G.D.; Stadtman, T.C.: Studies on the fermentation of *D*-α-lysine purification and properties of an adenosine triphosphate regulated B_{12}-coenzyme-dependent *D*-α-lysine mutase complex from *Clostridium sticklandii.* Biochemistry, N.Y. *9:* 4890–4900 (1970).

31 Horne, D.W.; Broquist, H.P.: Role of lysine and ε-*N*-trimethyl lysine in carnitine biosynthesis. J. biol. Chem. *248:* 2170–2175 (1973).

32 Bremer, J.: Carnitine precursors in the rat. Biochim. biophys. Acta *57:* 327–335 (1962).

33 Lindstedt, G.; Lindstedt, S.: Studies on the biosynthesis of carnitine. J. biol. Chem. *240:* 316–321 (1965).

34 Broquist, H.P.: Carnitine biosynthesis in *Neurospora crassa;* in Fraenkel, McGarry,

Carnitine biosynthesis, metabolism and functions, pp. 7–17 (Academic Press, New York 1980).

35 Borum, P.R.; Broquist, H.P.: Purification of *S*-adenosyl methionine, ε-*N*-*L*-lysine methyl transferase. The first enzyme of carnitine biosynthesis. Biol. Chem. *252:* 5651–5655 (1977).

36 Durban, E.; Nochumson, S.; Kim, S.; Paik, W.K.; Shung, K.C.: Cytochrome *c*-specific protein-lysine methyl transferase from *Neurospora crassa.* J. biol. Chem. *253:* 1427–1435 (1978).

37 Paik, W.K.; Kim, S.: Solubilization and partial purification of protein methylase III from calf thymus nuclei. J. biol. Chem. *245:* 6010–6015 (1970).

38 Labadie, J.; Dunn, W.A.; Aronson, N.N.: Hepatic synthesis of carnitine from protein-bound trimethyl-lysine. Lysosomal digestion of methyl-lysine-labelled asialo fetuin. Biochem. J. *160:* 85–95 (1976).

39 Khan-Siddiqui, L.; Bamji, M.S.: Lysine-carnitine conversion in normal and undernourished adult men – suggestion of a nonpeptidyl pathway. Am. J. clin. Nutr. *37:* 93–98 (1983).

40 ElAmin, B.; Means, G.E.: Introduction of methyl groups from ε-*N*-methyl lysine into the one-carbon pool. Biochem. biophys. Res. Commun. *86:* 407–414 (1970).

41 Rebouche, C.J.: Comparative aspects of carnitine biosynthesis in microorganisms and mammals with attention to carnitine biosynthesis in man; in Fraenkel, McGarry, Carnitine biosynthesis, metabolism and functions, pp. 57–72 (Academic Press, New York 1980).

42 Hoppel, C.L.; Novak, R.; Cox, R.A.: 6-*N*-Trimethyl lysine metabolism and carnitine biosynthesis (Abstract). Fed. Proc. *35:* 1478 (1976).

43 Hochalter, J.B.; Henderson, L.M.: Carnitine biosynthesis: the formation of glycine from carbons 1 and 2 of 6-*N*-trimethyl-*L*-lysine. Biochem. biophys. Res. Commun. *70:* 364–366 (1976).

44 Kaufman, R.A.; Broquist, H.P.: Biosynthesis of carnitine in *Neurospora crassa.* J. biol. Chem. *252:* 7437–7439 (1977).

45 Haigler, H.T.; Broquist, H.P.: Carnitine synthesis in rat tissue slices. Biochem. biophys. Res. Commun. *56:* 676–681 (1974).

46 Carter, A.L.; Frenkel, R.: The role of kidney in the biosynthesis of carnitine in the rat. J. biol. Chem. *254:* 10670–10674 (1979).

47 Zaspel, B.J.; Sheridan, K.J.; Henderson, L.M.: Transport and metabolism of carnitine precursors in various organs of the rat. Biochim. biophys. Acta *631:* 192–202 (1980).

48 Rebouche, C.J.; Engel, A.G.: Tissue distribution of carnitine biosynthetic enzymes in man. Biochim. biophys. Acta *630:* 22–29 (1980).

49 Rebouche, C.J.; Engel, A.G.: Significance of renal gamma-butyrobetaine hydroxylase for carnitine biosynthesis in man. J. biol. Chem. *255:* 8700–8705 (1980).

50 Paik, W.K.; Kim, S.: in Protein methylation, pp. 112–141 (Wiley, New York 1980).

51 Hulse, J.D.; Ellis, S.R.; Henderson, L.M.: Carnitine biosynthesis, β-hydroxylation of trimethyl lysine by an α-ketoglutarate dependent mitochondrial dioxygenase. J. biol. Chem. *253:* 1654–1657 (1978).

52 Henderson, L.M.; Hulse, J.D.; Henderson, L.L.: Purification of the enzymes involved in the conversion of trimethyl lysine to trimethyl aminobutyrate; in Fraenkel,

McGarry, Carnitine biosynthesis, metabolism and functions, pp. 35–43 (Academic Press, New York 1980).

53 Hulse, J.D.; Henderson, L.M.: Carnitine biosynthesis: purification of 4-*N*-trimethyl aminobutyraldehyde dehydrogenase from beef liver. J. biol. Chem. *255:* 1146–1151 (1980).

54 Lindstedt, G.; Lindstedt, S.; Nordin, I.: Hydroxylation of γ-butyrobetaine; in Fraenkal, McGarry, Carnitine biosynthesis, metabolism and functions, pp. 45–56 (Academic Press, New York 1980).

55 Englard, S.; Carnicero, H.H.: γ-Butyrobetaine hydroxylation to carnitine in mammalian kidney. Archs Biochem. Biophys. *190:* 361–364 (1978).

56 Englard, S.: Hydroxylation of γ-butyrobetaine to carnitine in human and monkey tissues. FEBS Lett. *102:* 297–300 (1979).

57 Sachan, D.S.; Broquist, H.P.: Synthesis of carnitine from epsilon-*N*-trimethyl lysine in post mitochondrial fractions of *Neurospora crassa.* Biochem. biophys. Res. Commun. *96:* 870–875 (1980).

58 Mitchell, M.E.: Carnitine metabolism in human subjects. I. Normal metabolism. Am. J. clin. Nutr. *31:* 293–306 (1978).

59 Travassos, L.R.; Sales, C.O.: Microbiological assay of carnitine. Analyt. Biochem. *58:* 485–499 (1974).

60 Lewin, L.M.; Peshin, A.; Sklarz, B.: A gas chromatographic assay for carnitine. Analyt. Biochem. *68:* 531–536 (1975).

61 Pearson, D.J.; Tubbs, P.K.: Carnitine and derivatives in rat tissues. Biochem. J. *105:* 953–963 (1967).

62 Brooks, D.E.; McIntosh, J.E.A.: Turnover of carnitine by rat tissues. Biochem. J. *148:* 439–445 (1975).

63 Tsai, A.C.; Romsos, D.R.; Leveille, C.A.: Significance of dietary carnitine for growth and carnitine turnover in rats. J. Nutr. *104:* 782–792 (1974).

64 Cederblad, G.; Lindstedt, S.: Metabolism of labelled carnitine in the rat. Archs Biochem. Biophys. *175:* 173–180 (1976).

65 Khairallah, E.A.; Wolf, G.: Carnitine decarboxylase. The conversion of carnitine to β-methylcholine. J. biol. Chem. *242:* 32–39 (1967).

66 Borum, P.R.: Regulation of carnitine concentration in plasma; in Fraenkel, McGarry, Carnitine biosynthesis, metabolism and functions, pp. 115–126 (Academic Press, New York 1980).

67 Mitchell, M.E.: Carnitine metabolism in human subjects. II. Values of carnitine in biological fluids and tissues of 'normal' subjects. Am. J. clin. Nutr. *31:* 481–491 (1978).

68 Pace, J.A.; Wannemacher, R.W., Jr.; Neufeld, H.A.: Improved radiochemical assay for carnitine and its derivatives in plasma and tissue extracts. Clin. Chem. *24:* 32–35 (1978).

69 Hoppel, C.; Genuth, S.; Brass, E.; Fuller, R.; Hostetler, K.: Carnitine and carnitine palmitoyltransferase; in Fraenkel, McGarry, Carnitine biosynthesis, metabolism and functions, pp. 287–305 (Academic Press, New York 1980).

70 Askew, E.W.; Hecker, A.L.; Wise, W.R.: Dietary carnitine and adipose tissue turnover rate in exercise trained rats. J. Nutr. *107:* 132–142 (1977).

71 Borum, P.R.; Broquist, H.P.: Lysine deficiency and carnitine in male and female rats. J. Nutr. *107:* 1209–1215 (1977).

72 Khan, L.; Bamji, M.S.: Tissue carnitine deficiency due to dietary lysine deficiency: triglyceride accumulation and concomitant impairment in fatty acid oxidation. J. Nutr. *109:* 24–31 (1979).

73 Tanphaichitr, V.; Zaklama, M.S.; Broquist, H.P.: Dietary lysine and carnitine: relation to growth and fatty livers in rats. J. Nutr. *106:* 111–117 (1976).

74 Taylor, M.J.; Stapleton, P.: Effect of maternal dietary lysine deficiency on tissue carnitine levels in the rat (Abstract). Fed. Proc. *39:* 1045 (1980).

75 Chu, S.W.; Hegsted, D.M.: Adaptive response of lysine and threonine degrading enzymes in adult rats. J. Nutr. *106:* 1089–1096 (1976).

76 Tanphaichitr, V.; Horne, D.W.; Broquist, H.P.: Lysine: a precursor of carnitine in the rat. J. biol. Chem. *246:* 6364–6366 (1971).

77 Khairallah, E.A.; Wolf, G.: Growth-promoting and lipotropic effect of carnitine in rats fed diets limited in protein and methionine. J. Nutr. *87:* 469–476 (1965).

78 Wilhelmus, I.S.; Waslien, C.; Broquist, H.P.; quoted by Broquist, H.P.; Borum, P.R.: Some aspects of carnitine nutriture. Compreh. Ther. *3:* 66–72 (1977).

79 Khan, L.; Bamji, M.S.: Plasma carnitine levels in children with protein-calorie malnutrition before and after rehabilitation. Clinica chim. Acta *75:* 163–166 (1977).

80 Khan-Siddiqui, L.; Bamji, M.S.: Plasma carnitine levels in adult males in India: effects of high cereal low fat diet, fat supplementation and nutrition status. Am. J. clin. Nutr. *33:* 1259–1263 (1980).

81 Mikhail, M.M.; Mansour, M.M.: The relationship between serum carnitine levels and the nutritional status of patients with schistosomiasis. Clinica chim. Acta *71:* 207–214 (1976).

82 Konig, B.; McKaigney, E.; Conteh, S.; Ross, B.: Effect of a lipid load on blood and urinary carnitine in man. Clinica chim. Acta *88:* 121–125 (1978).

83 Seccombe, D.W.; Hahn, P.; Novak, M.: The effect of diet and development on blood levels of free and esterified carnitine in the rat. Biochim. biophys. Acta *528:* 483–489 (1978).

84 Tanphaichitr, V.; Lerdvuthisopon, N.; Dhanamitta, S.; Broquist, H.P.: Carnitine status in Thai adults. Am. J. clin. Nutr. *33:* 876–880 (1980).

85 Symthe, P.M.; Swaneoel, A.; Campbell, J.A.H.: The heart in kwashiorkor. Br. med. J. *i:* 67–73 (1962).

86 Hughes, E.E.; Hurley, R.J.; Jones, E.: Dietary ascorbic acid and muscle carnitine in guinea pigs. Br. J. Nutr. *43:* 385–387 (1980).

87 Nelson, P.J.; Pruitt, R.E.; Henderson, L.L.; Jenness, R.; Henderson, L.M.: Effect of ascorbic acid deficiency on the in vivo synthesis of carnitine. Biochim. biophys. Acta *672:* 123–127 (1981).

88 Dunn, W.A.; Aronson, N.N., Jr.; Englard, S.: The effects of *l*-amino-*D*-proline on the production of carnitine from exogenous protein-bound trimethyl lysine by perfused liver. J. biol. Chem. *257:* 7948–7951 (1982).

89 Corredor, C.; Mansbach, C.; Bressler, R.: Carnitine depletion in choline-deficient state. Biochim. biophys. Acta *144:* 366–374 (1967).

90 Scholte, H.R.; Stinis, J.T.; Jennekens, F.G.I.: Carnitine levels in pregnancy. New Engl. J. Med. *299:* 1079–1080 (1978).

91 Hahn, P.; Skala, J.P.; Seccombe, D.W.; Frohlich, J.; Penn-Walker, D.; Novak, M.; Hynie, I.; Towell, M.E.: Carnitine content of blood and amniotic fluid. Pediat. Res. *11:* 878–880 (1977).

92 Schmidt-Sommerfeld, E.; Novak, M.; Penn, D.; Wieser, P.B.; Buch, M.; Hahn, P.: Carnitine and development of new-born adipose tissue. Pediat. Res. *12:* 660–664 (1978).
93 Novak, M.; Monkus, E.F.; Chung, D.; Buch, M.: Carnitine in the perinatal metabolism of lipids. I. Relationship between maternal and fetal plasma levels of carnitine and acyl carnitines. Pediatrics, Springfield *67:* 95–100 (1981).
94 Borum, P.R.; York, C.M.; Broquist, H.P.: Carnitine content of liquid formulas and special diets. Am. J. clin. Nutr. *32:* 2272–2276 (1979).
95 Novak, M.; Wieser, P.B.; Buch, M.; Hahn, P.: Acetyl carnitine and free carnitine in body fluids before and after birth. Pediat. Res. *13:* 10–15 (1979).
96 Wieser, P.B.; Buch, M.; Novak, M.: Effect of carnitine on ketone body production in human newborns (Abstract). Pediat. Res. *12:* 401 (1978).
97 Curry, E.; Warsaw, J.B.: Higher serum carnitine levels and ketogenesis in breast-fed as compared to formula-fed infants (Abstract). Pediat. Res. *12:* 504 (1978).
98 Rudman, D.; Sewell, C.W.; Ansley, J.D.: Deficiency of carnitine in cachectic cirrhotic patients. J. clin. Invest. *60:* 716–723 (1977).
99 Rudman, D., Ansley, J.D.; Sewell, C.W.: Carnitine deficiency in cirrhosis; in Fraenkel, McGarry, Carnitine biosynthesis, metabolism and functions, pp. 307–319 (Academic Press, New York 1980).
100 Chu, S.; Lincoln, S.D.: Increased serum carnitine concentration in renal insufficiency. Clin. Chem. *23:* 278–280 (1977).
101 Bohmer, T.; Bergrem, H.; Eiklid, K.: Carnitine deficiency induced during intermittent haemodialysis for renal failure. Lancet *i:* 126–128 (1978).
102 Battistella, P.A.; Angelini, C.; Vergani, L.; Bertoli, M.; Orenzi, S.: Carnitine deficiency induced during hemodialysis. Lancet *i:* 939 (1978).
103 Bizzi, A.; Cini, M.; Garattini, S.; Mingardi, G.; Licini, L.; Mecca, G.: *L*-Carnitine addition to hemodialysis fluid prevents plasma carnitine deficiency during dialysis. Lancet *i:* 882 (1979).
104 Bougneres, P.F.; Lacour, B.; DiGiulio, S.; Assan, R.: Hypolipaemic effect of carnitine in uraemic patients. Lancet *i:* 1401–1402 (1979).
105 Vacha, G.; Icardi, G.P.: Drug treatment of hypertriglyceridaemia in chronic uraemic patients: preliminary report on *D,L*-carnitine and thiadenol. Proc. Eur. Dial. Transpl. Ass. *17:* 367–371 (1980).
106 Guarnieri, G.F.; Ranieri, F.; Toigo, G.; Vasile, A.; Ciman, M.; et al.: Lipid-lowering effect of carnitine in chronically uraemic patients treated with maintenance haemodialysis. Am. J. clin. Nutr. *33:* 1489–1492 (1980).
107 Bazzato, G.; Mezzina, C.; Ciman, M.; Guarnieri, G.: Myasthenia-like syndrome associated with carnitine in patients on long-term haemodialysis. Lancet *i:* 1041–1042 (1979).
108 Engel, A.G.: Possible causes and effects of carnitine deficiency in man; in Fraenkel, McGarry, Carnitine biosynthesis, metabolism and functions, pp. 271–284 (Academic Press, New York 1980).
109 Broquist, H.P.; Borum, P.R.: Carnitine biosynthesis: nutritional implications; in Draper, Adv. Nutr. Res., vol. 4, pp. 181–204 (1982).
110 Rebouche, C.J.; Engel, A.G.: In vitro analysis of hepatic carnitine biosynthesis in human system carnitine deficiency. Clinica chim. Acta *106:* 295–300 (1980).

111 Wittels, B.; Bressler, R.: Biochemical lesion of diphtheria toxin in the heart. J. clin. Invest. *43:* 630–637 (1964).
112 Molsted, P.; Bohmer, T.: The effect of diphtheria toxin on the cellular uptake and efflux on *L*-carnitine. Biochim. biophys. Acta *641:* 71–78 (1981).
113 Suzuki, Y.; Kamikawa, T.; Yamazaki, K.: Protective effects of *L*-carnitine on ischemic heart; in Fraenkel, McGarry, Carnitine biosynthesis, metabolism and functions, pp. 341–352 (Academic Press, New York 1980).
114 Suzuki, Y.; Kabayashi, A.; Musumura, Y.; et al.: Myocardial carnitine deficiency in chronic heart failure. Lancet *i:* 116 (1982).
115 May, M.E.; Aftring, R.P.; Buse, M.G.: Mechanism of the stimulation of branched chain oxoacid oxidation in liver by carnitine. J. biol. Chem. *255:* 8394–8397 (1980).
116 Brooks, D.E.: Carnitine in male reproductive tract and its relation to the metabolism of epididymis and spermatozoa; in Fraenkel, McGarry, Carnitine biosynthesis, metabolism and functions, pp. 219–235 (Academic Press, New York 1980).
117 Carter, L.A.; Stratman, F.W.; Hutson, S.M.; Lardy, H.A.: The role of carnitine and its esters in sperm metabolism; in Fraenkel, McGarry, Carnitine biosynthesis, metabolism and functions, pp. 251–269 (Academic Press, New York 1980).

M.S. Bamji, PhMD, National Institute of Nutrition,
Indian Council of Medical Research, Jamai-Osmania P.O.,
Hyderabad 500 007 A.P. (India)

Subject Index